Vaccine
Research
and
Developments

Vaccine Research and Developments

Volume 1

edited by

Wayne C. Koff

Vaccine Research and Development Branch
Division of AIDS
National Institute of Allergy and Infectious Diseases
National Institutes of Health
Rockville, Maryland

Howard R. Six

Research and Development
Connaught Laboratories Inc.
Swiftwater, Pennsylvania

Marcel Dekker, Inc.   New York • Basel • Hong Kong

ISBN: 978-0-8247-8619-9

This book is printed on acid-free paper.

Marcel Dekker, Inc.
270 Madison Avenue, New York, New York 10016

Current printing (last digit):
10 9 8 7 6 5 4 3 2 1

PRINTED IN THE UNITED STATES OF AMERICA

Preface

The development and delivery of safe and effective vaccines for infectious disease control rank among the greatest achievements in the history of biomedical research and public health policy. The spectacular success stories of vaccines against poliomyelitis, smallpox, measles, mumps, rubella, diphtheria, tetanus, and pertussis provide elegant examples of the significant public health benefits from immunization research.

Several biomedical and political factors have recently converged to stimulate a significantly greater interest in vaccine development. The explosive growth in biotechnological methods, particularly in molecular biology, immunology, and virology, has provided the scientific community with novel research tools to exploit in the application of new and improved vaccines. Second, the emergence of new pathogens such as HIV, with its rapid global spread to pandemic proportions, has reinforced the importance of disease surveillance and prevention/control programs, and has provided the stimulus for greater resources in vaccine development. Third, the unprecedented gathering of the world's leaders at the Children's Summit (New York, September 1990) to pledge support to development of improved and more cost-effective vaccines to combat childhood infectious diseases provided added momentum to growing vaccine development efforts. Finally, during times of budgetary and fiscal restraints, Ben Franklin's old adage that "an ounce of prevention is worth a pound of cure" has gained renewed interest, as the pragmatic economic benefits of safe and effective vaccines have stimulated public health policymakers to consider the wisdom of accelerating programs in vaccine development.

The pace and growth of research and development efforts for vaccines against the broad spectrum of infectious diseases, coupled with future applications of vaccines in such areas as autoimmune diseases and malignancies, led to the concept of establishing a series of monographs to highlight research advances and public policy issues surrounding applications of immunization research. This first volume highlights recent technical advances in immunopotentiation and antigen presentation, strategies to develop contraceptive vaccines and improve bacterial vaccines, and recent developments from vaccine clinical trials including current public policy challenges to expedite vaccine development. Pat Pietrobon and Pat Kanda review the capacity of lipophilic components to chemically modify peptide and protein antigens and thereby augment the immunogenicity of such antigens. Anna Aldovini and Rick Young provide a brief review of recombinant technologies to express viruslike particles, and the potential of noninfectious packaging mutants to serve as prototype vaccines. James Tam reviews the multiple antigen peptide approach to provide a novel presentation system for peptide vaccines. Gary Ott and colleagues describe the use of muramyl peptides as vaccine adjuvants. Nancy Alexander reviews the current status and future prospects for contraceptive vaccines, and Neal Burnette offers perspectives for improving pertussis vaccines. Finally, John La Montagne and George Curlin provide a comprehensive update from recent vaccine clinical trials, and Bob Stein reviews the legal and policy aspects associated with developing HIV vaccines.

Advances in biotechnology will undoubtedly lead to the development of new and improved vaccines against a wide range of human pathogens. The merger of these technologies with novel strategies for accelerating clinical evaluation and distribution of safe and effective vaccines offers new frontiers for disease prevention. In an effort to provide a forum for reviewing significant advances in immunization research, and for addressing scientific and public policy challenges for moving candidate vaccines from the laboratory to the population, we have established this series of monographs. We thank the contributors to this first volume, with a special thanks to Dianne Broadhurst and Kerry Doyle for administrative and editorial support, and we look forward to highlighting other frontiers in vaccine development in the next volume.

Wayne C. Koff
Howard R. Six

Contents

Contributors

Anna Aldovini, M.D. Whitehead Institute for Biomedical Research and Department of Biology, Massachusetts Institute of Technology, Cambridge, Massachusetts

Nancy J. Alexander, Ph.D. * Director, Applied Fundamental Research, Jones Institute for Reproductive Medicine, Eastern Virginia Medical School, Norfolk, Virginia

Rae Lyn Burke, Ph.D. Associate Director, Virology, Chiron Corporation, Emeryville, California

W. Neal Burnette, Ph.D. Amgen Inc., Thousand Oaks, California

George T. Curlin, M.D. Deputy Director, Division of Microbiology and Infectious Diseases, National Institute of Allergy and Infectious Diseases, National Institutes of Health, Bethesda, Maryland

Patrick Kanda, Ph.D. Associate Scientist, Department of Virology/Immunology, Southwest Foundation for Biomedical Research, San Antonio, Texas

---

Current affiliation: Special Assistant for Contraceptive Research, Contraceptive Development Branch, National Institute of Child Health and Human Development, National Institutes of Health, Bethesda, Maryland.

John R. La Montagne   Director, Division of Microbiology and Infectious Diseases, National Institute of Allergy and Infectious Diseases, National Institutes of Health, Bethesda, Maryland

Gary Ott, Ph.D.   Principal Scientist, Chiron Corporation, Emeryville, California

Patricia J. Freda Pietrobon, Ph.D.   Research Manager, Biochemical Sciencies, Research & Development Department, Connaught Laboratories, Inc., Swiftwater, Pennsylvania

Robert E. Stein, LL.B.   Member, Blicker Futterman & Stein, and Adjunct Professor of Law, Georgetown Law Center, Washington, D.C.

James P. Tam   Associate Professor, Rockefeller University, New York, New York

Gary Van Nest, Ph.D.   Associate Director, Virology, Chiron Corporation, Emeryville, California

Richard A. Young, Ph.D.   Member, Whitehead Institute for Biomedical Research, and Professor, Department of Biology, Massachusetts Institute of Technology, Cambridge, Massachusetts

TECHNICAL ADVANCES IN VACCINE DEVELOPMENT

I

Lipopeptides and Their Effects on the Immune System
Use as Vaccine Components

Patricia J. Freda Pietrobon
Connaught Laboratories, Inc.
Swiftwater, Pennsylvania

Patrick Kanda
Southwest Foundation for Biomedical Research
San Antonio, Texas

INTRODUCTION

The development of new and improved vaccines composed of highly purified components requires delving into at least two basic technological areas. The first of these areas is directly related to the biology and chemistry of the infectious organisms against which a vaccine is being developed and includes studies into the biochemistry and immunology of these organisms. The results of investigations into these areas, as they relate to production of highly purified subunit vaccines, are the identification and isolation of the components responsible for protecting an individual following exposure to an infectious agent and, hopefully, the process and methods for preparing and characterizing these antigens on a routine basis. Ideally, the prospective protective antigen is highly purified and highly immunogenic. Unfortunately, this latter characteristic is not generally retained following purification. It is well recognized that chemically inactivated subunit vaccines, as well as purified polypeptide, peptide, or polysaccharide vaccines, are less immunogenic than their whole-cell counterparts. The practical implications of this decrease in immunogenicity may be observed in 1) the need to administer a higher dosage level of a subunit vaccine over its whole-cell counterpart, 2) the need to administer multiple doses of subunit vaccines, or 3) an observed decrease in efficacy of the subunit vaccine in a specific target (1-6). A consequence of this situation is the requirement to enhance the immunogenicity of these highly purified vaccine preparations.

The necessity to enhance the immunological competency of highly purified subunit vaccines thus leads us into a second technological area—that of adjuvants and immune potentiators. Among the most effective adjuvants used in laboratory animals are Freund's complete (FCA) and Freund's incomplete adjuvants (FIA), lipopolysaaccharides, and those containing bacterial products (wax D, trehalose dimycolate, lipid A, etc.). The immune potentiating abilities of these adjuvants to stimulate components of both humoral and cell-mediated immune responses may be linked to the lipoidal nature of these adjuvants (7-10). Due to their associated toxic properties, however, these agents are unacceptable for use in humans. At present, only aluminum-based adjuvants are licensed for use in human vaccination (11). Generally, these adjuvants have a history of safe usage in humans, but occurrences of adverse reactions have been reported (12-14). Aluminum hydroxide gel (alum) has been shown to have significant effects on increasing the potency and decreasing the reactogenicity of combined diphtheria, tetanus, and whole-cell pertussis vaccines in infants (15). Alum, however, has been found to be ineffective in inducing a delayed-type hypersensitivity (DTH) response (16).

Other experimental adjuvants have been investigated for their ability to potentiate a humoral or a cell-mediated immune response, or both (Table 1). In many instances, adjuvant efficacy has been found to be a function of the specific structure of the adjuvant under study as well as certain physicochemical characteristics of the antigen with which the adjuvant is being combined. Thus, the rationale design of new vaccines composed of highly purified antigens or synthetic peptides should actually be a codesign of antigen and adjuvant that considers the chemical characteristics of the antigen and adjuvant components necessary for eliciting the required protective immune response.

Table 1 Experimental Adjuvants Investigated for Use in Vaccine Development

Adjuvant	Reference
Muramylpeptides and analogs	
MDP	17-19
Murabutide	20,21
Threonyl-MDP	22
B30-MDP	23-26
MTP-PE	27-30
ISCOMS	31-36
Saponin	10,16,37,38
Quil A	39
Liposomes	40-43
Stearyl tyrosine	44,45
SAF-1	46-50
Pluronic block copolymers	51-56
Polymethylmethacrylate	57-63
Polyglucans	64
MAP	65,66

This chapter reviews the information available on a specific approach used in potentiating the immunogenicity of antigens. We concentrate on the use of lipoidal peptides and lipoidal protein antigens as immunogens, and how the chemical modification of these peptides and proteins into a more "surface-active" form influences their immunogenicity. The effect of adding lipophilic components to proteins and peptides on both the humoral and the cell-mediated immune response to specific antigens is reviewed. The chapter is not intended to be a review of vaccine adjuvants, but studies comparing the efficacy of lipoidal antigens with more traditional adjuvant systems, such as FCA, aluminum salts, and oil-in-water emulsions, are discussed where appropriate.

BACKGROUND STUDIES

In the late '60s and through the '70s, several investigators explored how the immune system was affected by the lipophilicity of a protein antigen or hapten. Observations had been made relative to the topographical localization of antigen within popliteal lymph nodes as a function of its lipid content, and also that many lipid-rich organisms and oil adjuvants homed to the same area of the lymph nodes. Looking at the in vitro digestion of sheep red blood cells (SRBCs) by macrophages over several different time periods and the subsequent ability of these cells to induce either antibody production or DTH response, Pearson and Raffel (67) observed a loss in antibody-stimulating capability but an increase in the ability to induce a DTH response with increased digestion of antigen by phagocytes. They attributed this observation to a decrease in the overall size of the immunogen and to the loss of epitopes necessary for the induction of antibody production. Parish (68) reported that chemical modification of SRBCs by either periodate oxidation or acetoacetylation also reduced the ability of SRBCs to stimulate antibody production and preferentially increased their ability to induce higher levels of DTH. This decrease or complete inhibition of antibody production was again attributed to the masking of essential epitopes on the surface of the SRBCs by the chemical modification procedure used. Tom (see Ref. 69 for review) additionally suggested that this switch from antibody inducer to preferential affector of the cellular immune system by both the phagocytized and the chemically modified particulate SRBC antigen complex was due to the creation of a more lipophilic (hydrophobic) or nonpolar antigen complex. Such a conclusion was consistent with the findings of Turk (70) that the induction of a DTH response was influenced by the amount of lipid contained within an antigen.

To more clearly address the questions raised about which physicochemical characteristics of an antigen influence its ability to induce a humoral antibody response versus a DTH response, and whether these characteristics can be linked to antigen localization within specific organs of the immune system, several experiments were performed. Coon and Hunter (71) described a system whereby a soluble antigen such as bovine serum albumin (BSA), which is a weak stimulator of components of the humoral immune system and antibody production and has limited effect on the cellular immune response when injected into guinea pigs without adjuvant, could be dramatically changed. A sustained DTH response and no detectable antibody response was observed when a modified BSA antigen was injected, without adjuvant, into guinea pigs. In these studies the BSA was modified by conjugation to a nonantigenic simple lipid such as dodecanoic acid. Whereas multiple injections of BSA (without adjuvant) induced antibody production in guinea pigs, induction of a DTH response was observed only when this protein antigen was injected with an oil adjuvant such as complete FCA. Following conjugation of the fatty acid to BSA and subsequent injection of the lipid-protein conjugate into guinea pigs, a potent and sustained DTH response was observed. The magnitude of the DTH response could be associated with the molar lipid-to-protein ratio used during the conjugation procedure. The DTH response was specific for the BSA, and no humoral or cell-mediated immune response was detected against the lipid passenger molecule. Using radioactively labeled ^{125}I-BSA, the authors reported localization of the native protein into the germinal centers of popliteal lymph nodes. In contrast, lipid-conjugated ^{125}I-labeled BSA was found to preferentially localize within the paracortex of lymph nodes, where it presumably was able to interact with thymus-associated cells (T cells) of the immune system.

Dailey and Hunter (72) also reported that lipid-conjugated haptens could be prepared that were capable of inducing a DTH response that was hapten-specific. There was no detectable antibody response to the hapten or to a protein carrier contained within the lipid-protein carrier-hapten complex. The DTH response could be induced whether the lipid was covalently coupled to the hapten or simply nonspecifically adsorbed through electrostatic interactions to the protein carrier present within the hapten-protein carrier-lipid complex. In the latter case, a cationic detergent, dimethyldioctaldecylammonium bromide (DDA), was used. Using radioactively labeled conjugates, both types of lipid-derivatized hapten-^{125}I-protein carrier conjugates were found to preferentially localize within the paracortical areas of the lymph nodes, while the non-lipid containing hapten-^{125}I-protein carrier complexes were found to localize within the germinal centers of the lymph nodes. Subsequent studies have demonstrated that the immune potentiating effects of DDA can be affected by the route of administration and the antigen dose (73). Additionally, co-administration of DDA with either chemically modified lymphoma cells or solubilized tumor antigens led to enhanced antitumor responses in mice in both an immunoprophylaxis and a chemoimmunotherapy model. This enhanced response was thought to be due to a specific association of the lipophilic tumor antigen with macrophages (74,75). The induction of a hapten-specific DTH response has also been demonstrated for liposome-incorporated haptens (76,77). The mechanism of uptake of haptenated liposomes by murine peritoneal exudate cells (PECs) cultured in vitro has been demonstrated to occur by phagocytosis, but the rate of uptake and the mode of degradation of internalized haptenated liposomes were influenced by their lipid composition (78).

The effects that chemical modification of a protein's surface has on an antigen's ability to bind antibody in vitro, to localize to areas of regional lymph nodes, or to function immunogenically either as an inducer of antibody production or as a stimulator of certain cellular immune responses

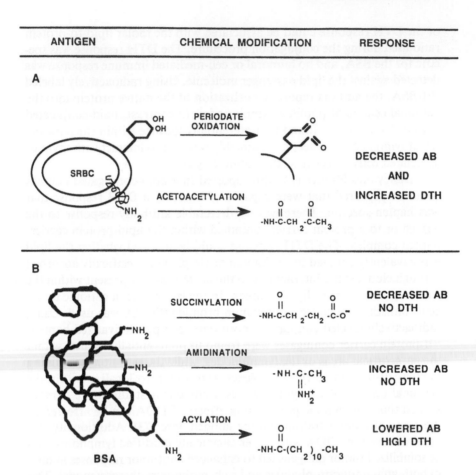

Figure 1 Effects on the immune response of chemical modification of antigens expressed on the surface of sheep red blood cells (A) and free amino groups of bovine serum albumin (B). In (A), periodate oxidation of surface carbohydrate is shown as an example, although a number of amino acids may also be oxidized. Lysine epsilon-amino and alpha-amino groups are affected primarily by aceto-acetylation. In (B), succinylation with succinic anhydride introduces negatively charged side chains primarily to lysine amino groups, amidination with ethyl-acetimidate alters the chemical structure of the positively charged side chain, and aceylation with dodecanoic anhydride attaches a hydrophobic tail to lysine amino groups, abolishing the positive charge and conferring lipophilic properties on BSA.

such as DTH were further studied by Coon and Hunter (79). In these studies, BSA was derivatized with either negatively charged succinyl groups or positively charged amidine moieties. This chemical derivatization did not affect the ability of these chemically modified BSA antigens to bind to anti-BSA antibody in a Farr-type radioimmunoassay. Derivatization of BSA with negatively charged succinyl groups completely suppressed

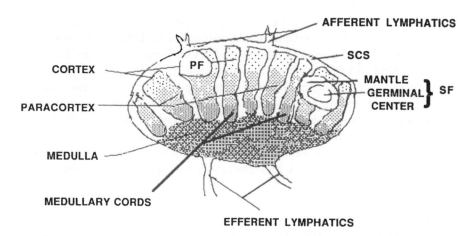

Figure 2   General structure of lymph node. The subscapular sinus (SCS) drains the extracellular space and is lined with phagocytic cells. The primary follicles (PF) lie directly under the SCS in the cortex of the lymph nodes and consist of small lymphocytes. The PFs become secondary follicles (SF) when germinal centers and mantle appear. A special form of reticular cells, the dendritic reticular cells which are capable of fixing antigen at their surfaces, are found in the germinal centers along with macrophages and other small and large lymphocytes. The cortical region as well as the medullary cords are populated mainly by the bursa and bone marrow-derived lymphocytes, and are therefore designated B-cell (or T-independent) areas. The T-dependent areas of lymph nodes are concentrated mainly in the paracortical regions. Here, APCs as interdigitating cells are believed to present antigen to T lymphocytes; hence the region is called the T-dependent area of lymph nodes. Investigations with ^{125}I-labeled proteins have shown that native (non-lipid-conjugated proteins) or chemically modified proteins preferentially localized within the germinal centers (B-dependent areas), while lipid-derivatized ^{125}I-labeled protein or hapten-protein conjugates homed to the paracortical regions of the lymph nodes, where they presumably associated with T lymphocytes.

the immunological response normally observed in guinea pigs to native BSA, even after multiple injections of the modified BSA. This suppression of the immunological response included both the serum antibody response and the lack of a BSA-specific DTH response.

Derivatization of BSA with positively charged amidine moieties had slightly different effects, including an increase in the serum anti-BSA antibody response normally observed to native BSA in guinea pigs and no detectable DTH response. On the other hand, when BSA was conjugated with long-chain (dodecanoyl) uncharged fatty acid groups, a strong BSA-specific DTH response was observed in guinea pigs, but, as previously reported, very little anti-BSA antibody was detected. Surprisingly, all three of these chemically modified BSA antigens showed similar abilities to bind anti-BSA antibody in vitro (Figure 1). Evaluation of ^{125}I-labeled antigen deposition within lymph nodes (popliteal, inguinal, and axillary) of previously unimmunized guinea pigs at 6, 24, or 96 hours postinjection showed that substantially more of the dodecanoyl-^{125}I-BSA persisted within the lymph nodes of these animals at all three time periods than did the two other chemically modified ^{125}I-BSA antigens. By 96 hours, succinyl and amidinated ^{125}I-BSA had essentially disappeared from the lymph nodes. In contrast, the lipoidal ^{125}I-BSA persisted in the medulla and remained substantially localized within the paracortical region of the lymph nodes (Figure 2).

The results observed for lipid-derivatized BSA were further extended for a second antigen, the purified protein derivative (PPD) of tubercle bacilli (80). Increasing the lipophilicity of PPD led to a PPD-specific DTH reaction in guinea pigs. These results, along with those observed for lipoidal BSA, supported the hypothesis that lipid-derivatized antigens can elicit specific cell-mediated T-cell-dependent DTH reactions without the aid of adjuvants.

EFFECT OF ANTIGEN LIPOPHILICITY ON CELLULAR INTERACTIONS

So far, we have discussed early studies employing either lipid-derivatized haptens or lipoidal proteins. These investigations demonstrated that as the lipophilicity of the antigens was increased, a specific T-cell-mediated immune response could be preferentially evoked by these antigens. Questions relating to the specific immunological mechanisms responsible for this altered immune response could then be addressed.

A series of experiments was performed that suggested that the stimulation of a cellular immune response by lipophilic antigens could be attributed to increased association of lipoidal antigens with cell surfaces (81), and that this association may be linked to the increased ability of these lipoidal antigens to associate with specific I-region gene products on the surface of antigen-presenting cells. Previous in vitro studies demonstrated a 25- to 50-fold greater uptake of lipoidal BSA by macrophages present within PEC than was recorded for the more hydrophilic non-derivatized BSA (82). Using autoradiography, localization of ^{125}I-labeled BSA within the draining lymph nodes of guinea pigs previously injected with lipid-derivatized BSA, amidinated BSA, or native BSA was studied. The lipophilic BSA was found to associate predominantly with macrophages within the medullary and paracortical areas of the lymph nodes. BSA modified by the covalent attachment of positively charged amidine groups had a somewhat decreased capacity to bind anti-BSA antibodies, as did lipoidal BSA, but, unlike the lipid-conjugated BSA, amidinated BSA did not stimulate a DTH response. Consistently, ^{125}I-labeled amidinated BSA was not taken up by macrophages within the lymph nodes.

In addition to the effects that lipid derivatization can have on the ability of a hapten or protein antigen to stimulate either a humoral or a cell-mediated immune response, lipid modification of certain adjuvants has also been shown to be effective in altering an adjuvant's antibody-stimulating or cell-mediated immune potentiating capabilities. N-acetyl-muramyl-L-alanyl-D-isoglutamine [muramyl dipeptide (MDP)] has been shown to be the minimal structural unit from bacterial cell walls that is capable of adjuvant activities (17). Utilization of MDP as an adjuvant in the aqueous form was found to potentiate the humoral antibody response to ovalbumin in guinea pigs. An increase in the antiovalbumin antibody response and induction of a DTH response was observed when both MDP and the protein antigen were coadministered in FIA. When MDP was conjugated with lipid moieties, it was able to induce DTH in the absence of FIA (83). In addition, increases in the ability of MDP to act as a nonspecific immunostimulator of protein antigens (84) and to enhance resistance to infection (23) were observed following lipid conjugation. These functions were related to the increased lipophilicity of MDP following conjugation to specific lipid components. Enhanced potentiation was observed when the lipophilic MDP, in saline, was administered to guinea pigs. This adjuvant activity could be further increased when certain lipid derivatives of MDP were incorporated within liposomes (27, 85).

Subsequent studies have shown that MDP can stimulate, both in vivo and in vitro, several functions of macrophages. These include the production of endogenous pyrogens, lymphocyte-activating factor, differentiation-inducing factor (D factor), and colony-stimulating factor (see Refs. 18 and 19 for review). Studies with two specific MDP derivatives—murabutide (21) and N-acetylmuramyl-L-threonyl-D-isoglutamine (threonyl-MDP) (22)—have shown that the adjuvant effects of the MDP class of adjuvants can be related to their ability to stimulate IL-1 production and to elicit production of lymphocyte growth factors (46-49). In the case of threonyl-MDP, this IL-1 activity is distinct from endogenous pyrogen.

Similar structure/function relationships have been investigated for a lauric acid conjugate of a tetrapeptide (LTP) isolated from crude immunostimulating extracts from *Streptomyces stimulosus* (86-88). The authors concluded from their studies that the immune potentiating properties of LTP were related to its amphipathicity, and that the lipophilic tail of LTP directed the binding of LTP to membranes of macrophages and/or lymphocytes.

ANTIGEN PRESENTATION AND THE INDUCTION OF SPECIFIC HUMORAL AND CELL-MEDIATED IMMUNE RESPONSES

Humoral and Cellular Interactions

In 1972, Parish (89) suggested that an inverse relationship existed between humoral and cell-mediated immunity that was mutually antagonistic. Since then, a remarkable number of discoveries made over the past 15 to 20 years show how the humoral and cellular components of the immune system actually work in concert to provide protective immunity. An important aspect of this interaction takes place on the cellular level and involves numerous cells of the immune system as well as costimulatory signals produced by these cells (90). Stimulation of CD4 helper and suppressor T lymphocytes and CD8 cytotoxic T lymphocytes requires that antigen be presented to these cells by other cells that take up the antigen. These cells are called antigen-presenting cells (APCs) (91). Both B cells and cells of the macrophage lineage can act as APCs (reviewed in Ref. 92). Observations from many laboratories have suggested that different APC populations present antigen with varying levels of efficiency (95,96). Nonetheless, antigen presentation to T cells is carried out by the APCs through transmembrane proteins present on the surface of the APCs. These antigens constitute what is termed the major histocompatibility complex (MHC). These glycoproteins are Ia gene products and form a bimolecular complex with antigen on the surface of the APCs such that presentation to either CD4 or CD8 T lymphocytes occurs in an MHC-restricted fashion.

Antigen presentation to CD8 cytotoxic T cells occurs in association with class I MHC molecules, while antigen presentation to CD4 T-helper and -suppressor cells occurs in association with the MHC class II glyco-proteins. T-cell stimulation then results from the interaction of the bimolecular antigen-MHC complex and the T-cell receptor (TcR) molecules on the surface of the T cells along with other costimulatory signals and putative adhesion ligands (non-MHC molecules) on the cell surfaces (Figure 3). Model phospholipid bilayer membranes have been used in a number of in vitro studies to investigate the interactions between the MHC

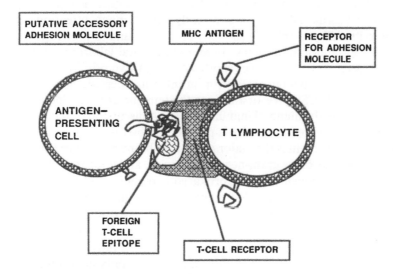

Figure 3 Schematic representation of interaction between APC and T lymphocyte. Foreign antigen forms a bimolecular complex with the ectodomain of MHC class I or class II antigens. This bimolecular complex on the APC is needed to interact with the TcR on T lymphocytes. It is believed that putative accessory adhesion molecules (non-MHC molecules) present on the APC surface, and costimulatory signals are required for T-cell activation and lymphokine production.

molecules and foreign antigens with the TcR molecules (97-103). Using artificial phospholipid vesicles reconstituted with either H-2 histocompatibility antigens from the mouse or HLA-A and HLA-B antigens from humans, the specificity of these interactions and some physicochemical characteristics of the ternary complex were elucidated, although antigen presentation by reconstituted liposomes was less efficient than that observed with glutaraldehyde-fixed APCs. The binding of peptides to class II MHC molecules in detergent solutions could be enhanced by certain lipids and their fatty acid composition (104).

Effects of Lipoidal Antigens on the Humoral Antibody Response

P_3CSS

Structure: Several groups of investigators have reported observations on the enhancing effects that conjugation of lipoidal components to protein and peptide antigens has on the humoral antibody response. One such compound, N-palmitoyl-S-[(2RS)-2,3-bis(palmitoyloxy)propyl]-cysteinyl-seryl-serine (P_3CSS), has recently drawn much attention. In addition to its ability to enhance antibody production and to protect guinea pigs from foot-and-mouth disease in an experimental laboratory model (105,106), Deres et al. (107) have reported on the in vivo priming of virus-specific cytotoxic T lymphocytes with an influenza peptide-lipopeptide construct of the P_3CSS. We first discuss the immune potentiating effect that P_3CSS has on the humoral immune system. A discussion of the P_3CSS effects on cell-mediated immunity is presented subsequently.

Braun's lipoprotein is the major outer-membrane protein in *Escherichia coli*, as well as other gram-negative bacteria, and appears to be ubiquitous in the outer membrane of prokaryotic organisms (108). Biosynthesis of Braun's lipoprotein first involves the synthesis of a precursor prolipoprotein, which is later modified and processed into the mature lipoprotein through a distinct signal peptidase (109). The protein component of Braun's lipoprotein is covalently linked to a fatty-acid tail consisting of an N-acyl diglyceride-cysteine moiety. The fatty acids linked as esters to the glycerylcysteine moiety in Braun's lipoprotein are mainly palmitic acid (45%), palmitoleic acid (11%), *cis*-vaccenic acid (24%), cyclopropylenehexadecanoic acid (12%), and cyclopropyleneoctadecanoic acid (8%). The fatty acids linked as amides to the N-terminal amino group are mainly palmitic acid (65%), palmitoleic acid (11%), and *cis*-vaccenic acid (11%). The tertiary structure of the protein component within Braun's

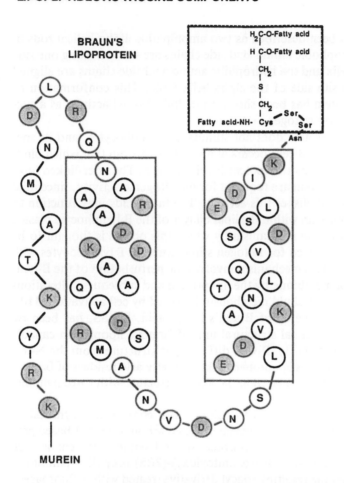

Figure 4 Schematic representation of Braun's lipoprotein and predicted secondary structure, with amino acid residues indicated in one letter code. The amino terminus comprises the N-acyl-S-diacylglyceryl-cysteinyl-seryl-serine moiety (dashed box), with the murein being attached to the ε-amino group of the carboxyl terminal lysine. The residues within the solid boxes are predicted to fold as amphipathic α-helices, based on circular dichroism measurements and Chou Fasman analysis (113). They are connected by a predicted β-turn region. The carboxyl terminal residues are arranged primarily as a β-sheet. The charged amino acids are shaded. In the synthetic P₃CSS analog of the N-terminus (dashed box), the fatty acyl moieties consist of palmitic acid.

lipoprotein has been described as two amphipathic alpha-helical rods in which the hydrophobic amino acid side chains are stacked along one side of the alpha-helix and the hydrophilic amino acid side chains are aligned along the opposite side of the alpha-helix (108). This conformation of Braun's lipoprotein has been shown to be linked to its activity as a specific B-lymphocyte mitogen.

Braun's lipoprotein does not stimulate T lymphocytes, and its specific interaction with B cells occurs at a site distinct from that which binds lipopolysaccharide, another potent B-cell mitogen. The ester-linked fatty acids of the lipoprotein are required for its mitogenic activity, since mild alkali hydrolysis abolishes this activity. The fatty acids may function to anchor the lipoprotein within the lipid bilayer of the B-lymphocyte plasma membrane (108). The mechanism by which this occurs is thought to be similar to that reported for mitogen stimulation of T lymphocytes with concanavalin A. This mechanism involves the perturbation of the B-lymphocyte plasma membrane by the lipoprotein and subsequent alterations in membrane phospholipid metabolism followed by cell activation (110).

The synthetic analog of Braun's lipoprotein, P_3CSS, has been reported to be the minimal structural unit of Braun's lipoprotein capable of adjuvant activity (111). P_3CSS differs in its structure from the N-terminal region of Braun's lipoprotein in that the fatty-acid residues of Braun's lipoprotein have been replaced in the P_3CSS structure with three palmitic-acid residues (Figure 4).

The seryl-serine portion of P_3CSS is most conveniently synthesized in solution phase using 9-fluorenylmethyloxycarbonyl (Fmoc)-based protection chemistry. The t-Butyl-protected seryl-serine fragment is then condensed with the S-[2,3-Bis(palmitoyloxy)-(2RS)-propyl]-N-palmitoyl-(R)-cysteine, and the resulting triacyl derivative treated with trifluoroacetic acid to yield the free P_3CSS (112). The synthesis is depicted in Scheme I.

The deprotected P_3CSS lipotripeptide can be purified by recrystallization from chloroform:methanol solutions at 0°. Lipopeptides of varying amino acid chain lengths are prepared by condensing the P_3C with protected peptide fragments prior to removing the amino acid side-chain protecting groups. Longer peptides (more than six amino acids) are more easily obtained by solid-phase synthesis, with the P_3C added onto the resin-bound peptide as the last step in the assembly. The completed lipopeptide is then treated with trifluoroacetic acid (TFA), which simultaneously cleaves the lipopeptide from the resin and removes amino acid side-chain protecting groups. Lengthening of the polar, peptidic portion of the lipopeptide often increases its amphiphilic character, resulting in

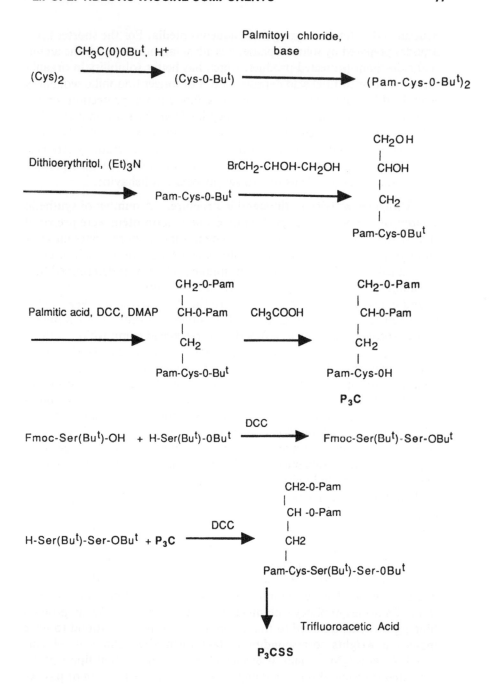

Scheme I

structures that tend to aggregate in aqueous media. For the shorter lipo-peptides prepared by solution phase, it is advantageous to purify the amino acid side-chain-protected product, which has better solubility in organic solvents, prior to final acid deprotection. For longer lipophilic sequences assembled by solid-phase synthesis using Fmoc-based protection, cross-linkers that allow cleavage of the lipopeptide from the solid support without concomitant side-chain deprotection should be employed (114). The protected lipopeptide segments are more easily separated from by-products in nonaqueous systems than the deprotected derivatives, which present unique solubility problems due to self-association behavior.

Mitogenic activity vs. lipopeptide structure: A number of synthetic analogs of the N-terminal portion of Braun's lipoprotein were prepared and studied for their abilities to stimulate murine B lymphocytes into im-munoglobulin secretion and for mitogenic activity toward spleen cells, as assessed by radioactive thymidine uptake (111). It was determined that the minimal structural requirement for a fully mitogenically active com-pound consisted of one serine linked to the P_3C derivative. Weak mito-genic activity was observed for the P_3C alone, but only at much higher doses. Mitogenic activity as a function of fatty-acid composition in these conjugates was also investigated (115). Murine polyclonal B-cell activa-tion in different inbred mouse strains was achieved after stimulation of their cultured spleen cells with N-palmitoyl-Ser-Ser-Asn-Ala. This com-pound could also stimulate murine B lymphocytes into immunoglobulin secretion (115). These effects were far less pronounced than those ob-tained using a tripalmitoyl-pentapeptide containing the P_3CSS, however (116). The tetrapeptide alone was only marginally active in these stud-ies, indicating the requirement for a lipophilic tail that may serve to anchor the mitogen in the lipid bilayer of the plasma membrane. Interaction with the lymphocyte plasma membrane was indeed demonstrated using a fluor-escently-labeled lipohexapeptide P_3C-Ser-$(Lys)_4$, which was able to induce capping and patching effects (117). Further association of these lipopep-tides with cell-surface receptors, MHC gene products, or membrane pro-teins involved in signal transduction would then be possible.

In support of this, P_3C was coupled to pore-controlled glass beads and used as an affinity column to bind radiolabeled membrane solubili-sates of murine lymphocyte plasma membranes (118). Specific lipoprotein-binding proteins adhered to this column, and some were found to have molecular weights corresponding to Ia-antigen, the δ-chain of cell sur-face IgD, and IgM μ-chain. It has also been speculated that lipopeptide-mediated transmembrane signaling may involve the activation of passive calcium channels (106). Since it is known that the interaction of many proteins with membranes is through the specific interaction of amphipathic protein secondary structural elements with phospholipids, it is of interest as to whether the presence of the triacyl moiety at the N-terminus of these lipopeptides can influence or induce these types of secondary structural features within the peptidic portions of these molecules. This phenomenon has been demonstrated experimentally with model lipid-associating-peptides bearing an N-terminal fatty acyl group, whereby the acylated sequences adopted α-helical structure upon binding to phospholipid bilayers (119). Similar findings were reported with basic amphipathic β-structural peptides upon interaction with negatively charged phospholipid bilayers (120). Physical studies of secondary structural changes within P_3CS-linked peptides following integration into model membrane systems may provide critical information pertaining to the contribution of the peptide portion toward mitogenic activity.

An interesting observation pertaining to the mitogenic properties of the P_3C derivatives focuses on the stereochemistry of the chiral center present at the glyceryl 2 carbon within the diacylglycerol moiety. The synthetic P_3CSS described by Wiesmuller et al. (112) incorporates the racemic 1-bromo-2,3-propanediol synthon in developing the s-diacylglycerol portion (Scheme 1). This yields a product comprising an equal mixture of two enantiomers, R,R and S,R, since the cysteine used is of the R configuration. Separation of these diastereomers revealed that the R,R isomer possessed much higher mitogenic activity than either the racemic (R,R; S,R) mixture or the S,R enantiomer. The R configuration at the glycerol 2 carbon is also found in naturally occurring membrane phospholipids. These findings suggest that simple intercalation of the lipoidal portion of P_3C-peptides into membrane bilayers may not be sufficient for optimal stimulation because the fatty acyl chains must have a specific orientation relative to the glyceryl backbone to interact effectively with membrane components. Although details of the synthesis of the R,R isomer of P_3CSS have not been reported, substitution of the optically active 3-iodoglycerol for the racemic 3-bromoglycerol yields the active isomer. The 3-iodo-*sn*-glycerol can be prepared from D-mannitol in a straightforward manner and serves to increase the accessibility of the active P_3C isomer (121,122).

Macrophage/monocyte stimulation by lipoidal peptides: It is known that macrophages play a key role in B-lymphocyte activation, although the precise mechanism(s) of this stimulation is unclear. Studies were conducted with two synthetic analogs of the N-terminal part of Braun's lipoprotein to determine if they could stimulate murine macrophages to activate B lymphocytes, and whether these lipopeptides could activate B lymphocytes directly in macrophage-depleted cultures (123). The lipoidal analogues P_3CS and P_3CSS-Asn-Ala were able to induce murine macrophages and human mononuclear cells to produce IL-1 in a manner similar to that found for bacterial lipopolysaccharide (LPS). P_3CSS-Asn-Ala was also able to induce the synthesis of prostaglandins E_2 and $F_{2\alpha}$ in murine peritoneal macrophages. Since IL-1 and prostaglandins are known to modulate the immune response and IL-1 can activate B lymphocytes, it appeared that lipopeptide stimulation of murine B lymphocytes might occur indirectly via macrophage activation. However, a residual lipopeptide-induced activation of BALB/c murine spleen cells persisted in adherent-cell-depleted cultures, demonstrating a direct interaction of the P_3CSS analogs with these cell populations.

The fate of various derivatives of P_3CS following incubation with murine bone-marrow-derived macrophages was determined using electron energy loss spectroscopy (EELS), a technique that allows monitoring of the subcellular distribution of these molecules (124). The results indicate that the intact P_3CS can migrate to different compartments within the cell and persist for considerable periods of time, suggesting that interaction of lipopeptides with intracellular components is important for macrophage activation. For instance, the diacylglyceryl portion may be released intracellularly as a metabolite, with the thiolated dipalmitoyl derivative functioning as a diacylglycerol (DAG) analog, which in turn can activate protein kinase C (PKC). Evidence exists for DAG activation of PKC to be an important step in the stimulation of different macrophage classes as well as quiescent B cells, and it has been suggested that LPS may act as a DAG analog in this capacity (125). Alternatively, protein receptors may exist within macrophages that can bind P_3CS at the surface and act as signal transducers. Specific macrophage receptors have been identified that recognize platelet-activating factor and LPS, which can initiate breakdown of polyphosphoinositides toward the generation of DAG (126). Phosphorylation of a variety of proteins by PKC evidently can lead to increased expression of certain mRNAs and consequent increased synthesis of specific proteins, prostaglandins, and IL-1.

In general, macrophage/monocyte cells are responsible for a broad spectrum of functions aside from activation of B lymphocytes, and are controlled by complex activation/inhibition pathways, many of them ill-defined. The potential role of lipoidal peptides in many of these processes remains largely unexplored.

Adjuvant activity of lipoidal peptides: Aside from its ability to function as a potent polyclonal B-cell mitogen and activator of macrophages, P_3CSS has also been shown to possess adjuvant activity. This was first demonstrated by a conjugate prepared with a synthetic peptide construct (amino acids 516-529) from the extracytoplasmic region of the receptor for epidermal growth factor (EGF-R) and an analog of P_3CSS, P_3CS (127). The P_3CS-EGF-R conjugate was administered as a single intraperitoneal injection to groups of three to five BALB/c mice, without additional adjuvants. Other groups within the study included noninjected control animals, the tetradecapeptide EGF-R 516-529 without adjuvant, P_3CS alone, and a mixture of EGF-R plus P_3CS. Antigen-specific ELISA antibody responses (IgG and IgM) were determined 14 days after immunization of the animals. An approximate 10-fold increase in the anti-EGF-R antibody titers was recorded when peptide was administered as a covalent conjugate with P_3CS. No potentiation of the antibody response was observed when peptide and P_3CS were administered as an admixed formulation. This suggested that covalent coupling of antigen to the tripalmitoyl glycerylcysteine-serine moiety is required for adjuvant activity. To achieve comparable antibody titers with a conventional peptide-BSA conjugate formulation, multiple injections in FCA were required. In vitro enhancement of antibody production in cell culture experiments was also demonstrated with the P_3CS-peptide conjugate.

The synthetic lipopentapeptide analog of P_3CSS, P_3Cys-Ser-Ser-Asn-Ala, was evaluated for its immune enhancing capabilities in vitro with particulate antigens such as underivatized SRBCs and a trinitrophenylated (TNP-) SRBC derivative (128). Adjuvant activity of the lipopentapeptide was evaluated in vitro in a direct hemolytic plaque assay. When assessing the in vitro primary immune response, antigen and lipopentapeptide, at varying doses of lipopentapeptide, were preincubated together for 1 hour at room temperature prior to being added to the cell cultures. The adjuvant effect of the tripalmitoyl pentapeptide was found to be dependent on the amount of lipopeptide added to the cell cultures. At optimal antigen and adjuvant doses (3.3 to 33.3 μg/ml lipopentapeptide), the number of plaque-forming cells in the cell culture was increased approximately 100 fold. A 10- to 60-fold increase in the number of plaque-forming cells was observed when suboptimal concentrations of the lipopeptide (0.03 to 0.3 μg/ml) were used. In order for immune enhancement to occur, antigen and adjuvant had to be added to the cell culture at the same time. No potentiation in the number of plaque-forming cells was observed if the tripalmitoyl pentapeptide was added to the cell cultures

1 day after antigen application. Administration of the lipopentapeptide 1 day before antigen was applied to the cell cultures even resulted in a significant decrease in the number of antigen-specific plaque-forming cells. These observations suggested that the immune enhancing effect of the tripalmitoyl pentapeptide could be due to a specific association between the particulate antigen and adjuvant. Evaluation of the supernatants from the cell cultures for the class of antibodies produced were performed by ELISA assays, specific for IgG and IgM. Both antigen-specific IgM and IgG responses were increased at least seven- and 10-fold, respectively. The magnitude of the enhanced IgG response over the amount of IgM antibodies produced suggested that the tripalmitoyl pentapeptide was capable of inducing antibody class-switching.

In a more recent study, the adjuvant activity of P_3CSS was demonstrated using a synthetic peptide construct VP1(135-154) from one of the four structural proteins of foot-and-mouth disease virus (FMDV) strain O_1K (105). In these investigations, outbred guinea pigs were immunized intramuscularly with a P_3CSS-VP1(135-154) conjugate emulsified in intralipid or liposomes. The efficacy of the lipopeptide and several other analogs of P_3C to protect guinea pigs following intradermal challenge with 500 guinea pig units of virulent FMDV 21 to 25 days after priming was compared. The criterion for protection was the absence of any secondary lesions for 10 days. One hundred percent (four of four) of the animals immunized intramuscularly with the P_3CSS-peptide conjugate were protected following live virus challenge. Protection ranged from 0 to 75% for the remaining experimental vaccines tested. The lipoidal vaccine appeared to be well tolerated by the guinea pigs, and no local reactions were observed after subcutaneous, intraperitoneal, or intramuscular injection of the tripalmitoyl-peptide-VP1(135-154) conjugate vaccine.

The effect of the stereochemistry of the s-glyceryl moiety of P_3CSS on adjuvant activity was also investigated (105,106). We noted earlier that the (R,R)-diastereomer of the N-terminal region of Braun's lipoprotein is a more potent B-cell mitogen than the (R,S)-diastereomer. Using a stereochemically pure preparation of (R,R)-P_3CSS, the dosage of (R,R)-P_3CSS-VP1(135-154) found to be effective in protecting guinea pigs following live virus challenge could be reduced to about one-half that used with an (R,R)-P_3CSS and (R,S)-P_3CSS mixed vaccine preparation. Circular dichroism analysis of the P_3CSS-VP1(135-154) vaccine revealed strong alpha-helical conformation for the FDMV peptide component attached to the palmitoyl tripeptide. This finding lends support to the importance of the presence of an alpha-helical structure to antigens involved in T-cell interactions. Prass et al. (129) have also demonstrated the importance of the attachment of at least one polar amino acid to the P_3C backbone for optimal B-cell stimulating activity. Thus, there are several physicochemical characteristics of the P_3CSS adjuvant that are responsible for its potent B-cell immune enhancing activities and its interactions with T lymphocytes and macrophages.

Lipoidal Antigens and Liposomes

The ability to design and modify the chemical structure of an adjuvant, relative to the physicochemical characteristics of highly purified antigens, may be essential to the development of efficacious subunit vaccines. Since the first demonstration of the adjuvant actions of liposomes in 1974 (42), liposomes have been shown to enhance the immune response in laboratory animals to haptenic (130) and multiepitopic antigens including polypeptide antigens such as HBsAg-derived polypeptides; detergent-extracted viral proteins from Semliki Forest virus, influenza virus, Epstein-Barr virus, measles virus, and herpes simplex virus (131,132); intact influenza virus, tetanus toxoid, allergens, many other protein antigens (41; for review see Ref. 43); and bacterial polysaccharide antigens and polysaccharide-protein conjugates (133). Recently, liposomes have been applied to detergent-extracted envelope glycoproteins from HIV-1 and evaluated for their enhancement to both humoral and cellular immune responses (134). Purified gp160/120 anchored into preformed liposomes as immunosomes induced high HIV-specific ELISA antibody titers (102,200 to 204,400) as well as high neutralizing antibody titers (320 to 640) when injected intraperitoneally into mice. Cellular responses, as measured by in vitro T-cell proliferation and by IL-2 production, were also enhanced by HIV immunosomes. Although the mechanisms responsible for enhanced immunogenicity displayed with liposomal adjuvants have not been fully defined, prolonged antigenic exposure due to increased retention of protein at the injection site and increased antigen delivery to macrophages by liposomes are thought to be major contributors to this phenomenon (135). In vitro studies have demonstrated that phagocytic engulfment of liposomes by macrophages is composition-dependent (136). Additionally, both the tumoricidal (137) and anti-infectious activity of liposomes bearing MDP were dependent on liposome type and on whether hydrophilic or lipophilic MDP was used (138).

A key factor to be addressed when formulating adjuvanted vaccines is maintenance of the native conformation of protein antigens such that relevant immunoprotective epitopes are presented properly to components of the immune system. Studies comparing different adjuvant systems with the same or different antigen preparations have shown that immune enhancement depends on the proper combining of antigen with adjuvant (31,139,140). Especially in the case of liposomes, enhancing capabilities can be improved by modifying the liposome type, size, lipid composition, or net surface charge (43,136,137,141,142) of specific formulations. Additionally, Therien and Shahum (143) have shown that a physical association between antigen and liposome is needed in order for enhancement of an antigen-specific humoral response by liposomal adjuvants to occur.

The flexibility and versatility with which liposomes can be prepared makes them an excellent system for studying adjuvant enhancing activities on the immune system with different antigens and peptides. Because liposomes consist of components that are biodegradable and immunologically inert, they have not been found to cause any significant local reactions and do not cause significant antigen accumulation in blood or internal organs (135). Liposomes have been safely administered into healthy human subjects with no significant adverse reactions reported (144). A Phase I safety trial recently initiated in normal healthy adults employs an experimental alum-adsorbed lipid A-containing liposome vaccine carrying a recombinant antigen, $R32NS1_{81}$, from the malaria circumsporozoite (R32) and the nonstructural protein (NS1) from influenza virus (145). Although the experimental vaccine contained high levels of monophosporyl lipid A (MPL), a nontoxic analog of lipid A, the vaccine appeared to be well tolerated by vaccinees following a single injection. IgG antibodies were detected against the repeating epitope from the malaria antigen within 2 weeks after the primary immunization, and these levels increased further following booster administration of the vaccine.

In addition to being able to modify the immune enhancing effects of liposomes by changing the lipid component and/or particle size, potentiation of the immune response may be further improved by covalent coupling of antigen to the liposome surface or by the inclusion of immunomodulators in liposomal formulations. Methods have been developed for the covalent coupling of antibodies (146-152), antigens (153-158), and sugars (159) to small unilamellar (SUV) and multilamellar (MLV) vesicles, making these antigens lipophilic in nature. Van Rooijen and Van Nieuwmegen (154) have shown no marked differences between the adjuvant effects of bovine gamma globulin (BGG) surface-coated liposomes and that of liposomes that have BGG (80%) entrapped within aqueous spaces between the phospholipid bilayers and surface-associated BGG (20%). From this the authors concluded that the enhancing effects of liposomes on the immune response were due to surface exposition of antigens. The enhancing effects of liposomes containing covalently coupled BSA were further increased by the entrapment of agents such as the enzyme inhibitor, methotrexate. Heath et al. (155) postulated that the liposomes used in the above study were able to bind to T-suppressor cells and that the entrapped methotrexate suppressed the proliferation of these cells, leading to enhanced antibody production.

This apparent enhancement of liposomal adjuvanticity through the surface association of antigens may, however, be linked to the physicochemical properties of the combined antigen-liposome formulations. Gregoriadis et al. (156) reported no statistically significant difference between the total IgG ELISA antibody response and the isotype distribution (measured as IgG1 and IgG2b) observed in BALB/c mice injected intramuscularly with tetanus toxoid entrapped in MLV dehydration-rehydration vesicles (DRV) or covalently coupled to DRV. In contrast to these findings, however, Shahum and Therien (157) observed a change in the antibody class distribution measured by a decrease in the ratio of IgG/IgM elicited by BSA-entrapped liposomes when three of four proteins tested were covalently linked to the surface of BSA-entrapped liposomes. The response observed with autologous protein covalently coupled to the surface of BSA-entrapped liposomes was similar to that elicited by liposomes bearing covalently coupled BSA on their surfaces. The authors suggested that this change in antibody class distribution by any surface-linked protein may be due to interactions between liposome-surface associated proteins and APCs.

Brynestad and colleagues (160-162) recently reported that the incorporation of a 23-residue peptide of glycoprotein D from herpes simplex virus type 1 (HSV-1) as an acyl-dipalmitic acid conjugate into liposomes increased both humoral and cellular immune responses in mice. When immunomodulators (MPL and/or MTP-PE) were included in the liposomal formulation, the humoral immune responses induced by the acyl-peptide-liposome constructs were greater than those induced by peptide in FCA. The isotype response to immunization was dependent on the particular antigen presentation system used. Acylpeptide-liposome constructs containing MTP-PE favored IgG_{2a}, which may be important in protection from viral infections.

The ability of liposomes to potentiate both humoral and cellular responses to peptide antigens is of considerable interest when developing purely peptide-based vaccines. Goodman-Snitkoff et al. (163) evaluated how the hydrophilicity and amphipathicity of a peptide influenced its ability to elicit an enhanced humoral antibody response following conjugation of the peptide to a lipid moiety and subsequent complexing of the lipoidal peptide with additional phospholipids to form liposomes. The authors reported that enhancement of an antibody response by lipopeptides incorporated within liposomes occurred when the peptide was amphipathic in nature and contained a putative B-cell epitope and a T-cell epitope. Antibody responses to nonimmunogenic hydrophilic peptides could be induced only if these peptides were presented in conjunction with an amphipathic lipopeptide phospholipid complex. Alternatively, enhancement of a humoral antibody response to hydrophilic peptides containing only putative B-cell epitopes could be achieved if peptides were conjugated to a lipid such as phosphatidylethanolamine (PE) and then incorporated into liposomes carrying either trace amounts of a detergent treated extract from Sendai virus or a peptide with putative T-helper cell determinants (164,165). The authors speculated that the formation of liposomes carrying lipoidal peptides containing putative B-cell and T-cell epitopes created a multivalent configuration of antigens that mimicked the natural presentation form of antigenic epitopes present in complex pathogens and thereby stimulation of both a humoral and a cell-mediated immune response (166). No direct measurements of enhancement to cellular components of the immune system were made, nor was the ability of these multivalent complexes to bind peptide-specific antibodies determined. Studies into these areas as well as others will be needed before the mechanism responsible for immune enhancement by these highly purified and synthetic peptide-lipid complexes is determined.

Lipopeptide Adjuvants and Cell-Mediated Immunity

We have discussed how humoral antibody responses to both protein and peptide antigens can be enhanced following their attachment to hydrophobic lipids. The degree of enhancement may be affected by physicochemical characteristics imparted to these lipoidal antigens by the chemical derivatization employed. This results in an altered capacity of these lipoidal antigens to interact with specific cells of the immune system. These alterations may include direct B-cell interaction and/or interaction with APCs leading to the stimulation of both T-helper and T-suppressor cells or CTLs. The processing and presentation of antigens to T-helper cells may be achieved by macrophages as well as B cells (167). Presentation by B cells favors activation of Th_2 cells, resulting in the production of predominantly IgG_{2a}, while presentation of antigen by macrophages favors activation of Th_1 cells and production of predominantly IgG_1 antibodies

(168,169). Using an in vitro antigen presentation system, Dal Monte and Szoka (158,170) have demonstrated that the topographical location of entrapped antigen versus lipoidal antigen presented on the surface of large unilamellar vesicles (LUV) affected whether antigen presentation was made by peritoneal macrophages or B-cell hybridoma cells. Encapsulation of pigeon cytochrome-c (PCC) into liposomes eliminated presentation by a B-cell hybridoma, yet it increased antigen presentation by macrophages as measured by interleukin-2 (IL-2) production. A 30- to 40-fold increase in IL-2 production over free PCC was observed when macrophages were used as presenting cells. B cells, however, could present lipoidal surface-bound PCC, but less efficiently than free PCC. When a synthetic peptide carrying a T-cell determinant of PCC was used as antigen with either live or glutaraldehyde-fixed peritoneal macrophages, both free and lipoidal surface-bound peptide stimulated IL-2 production. The surface-bound lipoidal peptide was a better inducer of IL-2 than was soluble PCC when live peritoneal exudate cells (PECs) were used as APC. Although the amount of IL-2 production induced by the liposome-incorporated lipoidal peptide was less than that observed with free peptide when glutaraldehyde-fixed PECs were used as APC, the results of these experiments demonstrate that lipopeptides presented on the surface of liposomes need not be processed by macrophages but can bind directly to Ia molecules and activate T-helper cells. These findings extend previously reported observations (171,172) that antigen processing need not occur with peptides carrying T-cell epitopes. These antigenic epitopes can bind to APC and then be presented to T lymphocytes in an MHC-restricted manner.

Studies by Brynestad and co-workers (160-162) have shown that incorporation of lipid-derivatized peptides into liposomes increased both humoral and cellular immune responses in mice. In these experiments, cellular immune responses were measured by lymphoproliferation and IL-2 production. Acylpeptide-liposome constructs containing lipoidal immunomodulators (e.g., MTP-PE) produced stimulation indexes (SI) equivalent to those observed with acylpeptide in FCA.

Deres et al. (107) have recently demonstrated the ability of two different lipopeptide derivatives of two of the major CTL epitopes from the nucleoprotein (NP) of influenza virus to prime virus-specific cytotoxic T lymphocytes in vivo in an MHC-restricted fashion. The experimental lipopeptide vaccines investigated were synthesized by conjugating a synthetic peptide corresponding to amino acids 147-158 (NP147-158) or amino acids 365-380 (NP365-380) from the influenza NP to P$_3$CSS.

By substituting the carrier portion of this conjugate with a nonproteinaceous lipid molecule, the phenomenon of epitope-specific suppression (173) observed with some protein-hapten conjugate vaccines may be avoided. The ability of the P$_3$CSS lipopeptide conjugates to prime influenza virus-specific CTLs in vivo was demonstrated to be MHC class I-restricted since only the CTLs from BALB/c mice (H-2d) could be primed in vivo following intravenous injection with P$_3$CSS-[NP147-158(R-)], an H-2d-restricted CTL-specific epitope, and (B6 × DBA/2) F1 mice (H-2b) responded only to the P$_3$CSS-NP365-380, an H-2b-restricted epitope from influenza NP.

In vitro studies incorporating detergent-solubilized Sendai virus protein and purified H-2 antigen into reconstituted membranes or liposomes demonstrated that soluble antigen presented in a hydrophobic environment could stimulate a MHC-restricted CTL response (174). These findings have been extended and include the observations that both soluble protein (175) and peptide fragments (176) can induce strong primary CTL responses in vitro. It was previously shown that class II-restricted T cells were stimulated by exogenous soluble proteins and that class I-restricted CTLs responded only to endogenously produced cellular antigens (92). Moore et al. (177) developed an in vitro model in which they could introduce exogenous antigen into target cells and stimulate a class I-restricted response. This was accomplished by the osmotic lysis of pinosomes (carrying the exogenous antigen), which released their contents into the cell cytosol. The released antigen was processed and found to associate with class I molecules. Thus, these investigations demonstrated that soluble antigen introduced into the appropriate intracellular compartment could be processed and presented in an MHC class I-restricted manner by target cells. Furthermore, Carbone and Bevan (178) showed that the ability of peptides to direct CTL recognition in vitro did not always persist in an in vivo priming model. They were, however, able to demonstrate that the synthetic peptide OVA(229-276) was capable of inducing in vivo a primary ovalbumin (OVA)-specific CTL response, after intravenous injection into C57BL/6 mice. The physicochemical characteristics responsible for the in vivo priming of class I-restricted CTL by OVA(229-276) were not clearly defined in these experiments. But Takahashi and colleagues (179) have shown that only a limited number of amino acid residues (in the immunodominant CTL epitope from the HIV-IIIB strain of the AIDS virus) are critical for binding of this AIDS peptide to class I MHC antigens, while other critical amino acids are needed for interaction with the TcR.

The above investigations suggest that a number of structural components (e.g., specific amino acid residues, lipid tails) and conformational characteristics (e.g., alpha-helix, amphipathicity, lipophilicity) influence whether an antigen can stimulate a class I- or class II-restricted response. In addition, the physicochemical characteristics responsible for in vitro target cell presentation may be different from those required for in vivo association of antigen with MHC antigens, as well as presentation to effector cells.

CONCLUSION

The development of improved, highly purified vaccines has certainly become a reality. As a result of advances made in recombinant DNA technology, synthetic peptide chemistry, adjuvant research, the development of models and algorithms for predicting B- and T-cell epitopes within an antigen, and a better understanding of how components of the immune system interact to elicit a humoral or cell-mediated immune response, vaccinologists now have access to "precision crafted tools" that can be used in the rationale design of efficacious vaccines. Investigations with totally synthetic lipopeptide constructs such as P$_3$CSS, or lipoidal proteins and peptides reconstituted into liposomes, have applied these tools with demonstrated efficacy in several animal protection models. What remains unclear, however, is whether there are any constitutive structural or conformational characteristics of an antigen that are required in order for chemical modification by lipophilic moieties to modulate and enhance an antigen-specific immune response. What importance does the presence of a B- or T-cell epitope play in the adjuvant action of lipopeptides and synthetically prepared chimeric lipoidal polypeptides? Investigations into the structure/function relationship and the mechanism of action of this unique class of adjuvants should provide the information needed so the rational design of vaccines incorporating synthetically constructed lipoidal antigens can be optimized and put into practical use.

ACKNOWLEDGEMENTS

We would like to thank Dr. William A. Hankins for reviewing this manuscript and Mrs. Joyce Moynihan for clerical support.

REFERENCES

1. Couch RB, Kasel JA, Pereira HG, Haase AT, Knight V. Induction of immunity in man by crystalline adenovirus type 5 capsid proteins. Proc Soc Exp Biol Med 1973; 143:905-908.

2. Kramp WJ, Six HR, Kasal JA. Postimmunization clearance of liposome entrapped adenovirus type 5 hexon. Proc Soc Exp Biol Med 1982; 169:135-139.

3. Melnick JL. Virus vaccines: an overview. In: Dreesman GR, Bronson JG, Kennedy RC, eds. High Technology Route to Virus Vaccines. Washington: American Society for Microbiology, 1985:1-14.

4. Warren KS. New scientific opportunities and old obstacles in vaccine development. Proc Natl Acad Sci USA 1986; 83:9275-9277.

5. Ada GL, What to expect of a good vaccine and how to achieve it. Vaccine 1988; 6:77-79.

6. Mitchell GF. The way ahead for vaccines and vaccination: symposium summary. Vaccine 1988; 6:200-205.

7. Warren HS, Vogel FR, Chedid LA. Current status of immunological adjuvants. In: Paul WE, ed. Annual Review of Immunology. Vol. 4. Palo Alto, CA: Annual Reviews, 1986:369-388.

8. Gall D. Observations on the properties of adjuvants. International symposium on adjuvants of immunity. Symp Ser Immunobiol Standard 1966; 6: 39-48.

9. Stewart-Tull D. Mineral oil adjuvants. Vaccine 1985; 3:152-157.

10. Bomford R. The comparative selectivity of adjuvants for humoral and cell-mediated immunity. Clin Exp Immunol 1980:435-441.

11. Edelman R. Vaccine adjuvants. Rev Infect Dis 1980; 2:370-383.

12. Wilson GS. The Hazards of Immunization. London: Athlone Press, 1967.

13. White RG, Coons AH, Connally JM. Studies on antibody production. III. The alum granuloma. J Exp Med 1955:102-73.

14. Turk JL, Parker D. Granuloma formation in normal guinea pigs injected intradermally with aluminum and zirconium compounds. J Invest Dermatol 1977; 68(6):336-340.

15. Butler NR, Voyce MA, Burland WI, Hilton ML. Advantages of aluminum hydroxide adsorbed combined diphtheria, tetanus, and pertussis vaccines for the immunization of infants. Brit Med J 1960; 1:663-666.

16. Bomford RHR. The differential adjuvant activity of Al(OH)₃ and saponin. In: Majde JA, ed. Progress in Leucocyte Biology: Immunopharmacology of Infectious Diseases. New York: Alan R Liss, 1987:165-170.

17. Ellouz F, Adam A, Giorbaru R, Lederer E. Minimal structural requirements for adjuvant activity of bacterial peptidoglycan derivatives. Biochem Biophys Res Comm 1974; 59(4):1317-1325.

18. Adam M. Muramylpeptides and analogues. In: Bona C, ed. Synthetic Adjuvants: Modern Concepts in Immunology. Vol 1. New York: John Wiley, 1985:1-58.

19. Audibert F, Leclerc C, Chedid L. Muramyl peptide as immunopharmacological response modifiers. In: Torrence PF, ed. Biological Response Modifiers: New Approaches to Disease Intervention. New York: Academic Press, 1985:307-327.

20. Telzak E, Wolfe SM, Dinarello CA, Conlon T, Kholy AE, Bahr GM, Choay JP, Morin A, Chedid L. Clinical evaluation of the immunoadjuvant murabutide, a derivative of MDP, administered with a tetanus toxoid vaccine. J Infect Dis 1986; 153(3):628-633.

21. Lefrancier P, Demier M, Jamet X, Choay E, Lederer E, Audibert F, Parant F, Parant M, Chedid L. A pyrogenic, adjuvant-active N-acetylmuramyl dipeptides. J Med Chem 1982:90-93.

22. Byars NE. Two adjuvant active muramyl dipeptide analogs induce differential production of lymphocyte-activating factor and a factor causing distress in guinea pigs. Infect Immunol 44:344-350.

23. Matsumoto K, Ogawa H, Kusama T, Nagase O, Sawaki N, Inage M, Kusumoto S, Shiba T, Azuma I. Stimulation of nonspecific resistance to infection induced by 6-O-Acyl muramyl dipeptide analogs in mice. Infect Immunol 1981; 32(2):748-758.

24. Kotani S, Kinoshita F, Morisaki I, Shimono T, Okunaga T, Takada H, Tsujimoto M, Watanabe Y, Kato K. Immunoadjuvant activities of synthetic 6-O-acyl-n-acetylmuramyl-L-alanyl-d-isoglutamine with special reference to the effect of its administration with liposomes. Biken J 1977; 20:95-103.

25. Tsujimoto M, Kotani S, Shiba T, Kusumoto S. Adjuvant activity of 6-O-acyl-muramyldipeptides to enhance primary cellular and humoral immune responses in guinea pigs: dose-response and local reactions observed with selected compounds. Infect Immunol 1986; 53(3):517-521.

26. Tsujimoto M, Kotani S, Okunaga T, Kubo T, Takada H, Kubo T, Shiba T, Kusumoto S, Takahashi T, Goto Y, Kinoshita F. Enhancement of humoral immune responses against viral vaccines by a non-pyrogenic 6-O-acyl-muramyldipeptide and synthetic low toxicity analogues of lipid A. Vaccine 1989; 7:39-48.

27. Ho RJY, Merigan TC. Antigen presenting liposomes as an adjuvant to enhance antigen mediated immunotherapy: Experience with recurrent disease of genital herpes simples virus type 2 infection in guinea pigs. Abstract. Conference in AIDS vaccine research, Second annual meeting of the national cooperative vaccine development groups for AIDS. October 15-18, 1989.

28. Ho RJY, Burke RL, Merigan TC. Antigen-presenting liposomes are effective in treatment of recurrent herpes simples virus genitalis in guinea pigs. J Virol 1989; 63(7):2951-2958.

29. Sanchez-Pescador L, Burke RL, Ott G, Van Nest G. The effect of adjuvants on the efficacy of a recombinant herpes simples virus glycoprotein vaccine. J Immunol 1988; 141:1720-1727.

30. Iido J, Saiki I, Ishihara C, Azuma I. Prophylactic activity against sendai virus infection and macrophage activation with lipophilic derivatives of N-acetylglycosaminylmuramyl tri- or tetrapeptides. Vaccine 1989; 7:225-228.

31. Morein B. Immunogenicity of different physical forms of viral antigenic subunits. In: Morrison WI, ed. Ruminant Immune System in Health and Disease. New York: Cambridge University Press, 1987:478-495.

32. Sundquist B, Lovgren K, Morein B. Influenza virus ISCOMs: antibody response in animals. Vaccine 1988; 6:49-53.
33. Morein B. The iscom antigen-presenting system. Nature 1988; 332:287-288.
34. Osterhaus A, Weijer K, UytdeHaag F, Knell P, Jarrett O, Akerblom L, Morein B. Serological responses in cats vaccinated with FeLV ISCOM and an inactivated FeLV vaccine. Vaccine 1989; 7:137-141.
35. Akerblom L, Stromstedt K, Hoglund S, Osterhaus A, Morein B. Formation and characterization of FeLV ISCOMs. Vaccine 1989; 7:142-146.
36. Pyle SW, Morein B, Bess JW Jr, Akerblom L, Nara PL, Nigida SM Jr, Lerche NW, Robey WG, Fischinger PJ, Arthur LO. Immune response to immunostimulatory complexes (ISCOMs) prepared from human immunodeficiency virus type 1 (HIV-1) or the HIV-1 external envelope glycoprotein (gp120). Vaccine 1989; 7:465-473.
37. Kensil CR. Adjuvant effect of purified saponins from Quillaja saponaria-dose response studies in mice. Abstract. International conference on advances in AIDS vaccine research, Third Annual Meeting of the National Cooperative vaccine development groups for AIDS. October 1-5, 1990.
38. Newman MJ. Saponin adjuvant induced enhancement of immune responses to an experimental recombinant HIV-1 env vaccine. Abstract. International conference on advances in AIDS vaccine research, Third annual meeting of the national cooperative vaccine development groups for AIDS. October 1-5, 1990.
39. Verheul AFM, Versteeg AA, DeReuver MJ, Jansze M, Snippe H. Modulation of the immune response to pneumococcal type 14 capsular polysaccharide-protein conjugates by the adjuvant quil A depends on the properties of the conjugates. Infect Immunol 1989; 57(4):1078-1083.
40. Gregoriadis G. Immunological adjuvants: a role for liposomes. Immunol Today 1990; 11(3):89-97.
41. Alving CR. Liposomes as carriers for vaccines. In: Ostro JM, ed. Liposomes from Biophysics to Therapeutics. New York: Marcel Dekker, 1987:195-218.
42. Allison AC, Gregoriadis G. Liposomes as immunological adjuvants. Nature (London) 1974; 252:252.
43. Six HR, Anderson C, Kasel JA. Further studies of liposomes as carriers of purified protein vaccines. In: Gregoriadis G, ed. Liposomes as Drug Carriers. Somerset: John Wiley, 1988:197-206.
44. Landi S, Penney CL, Shah P, Hart F, Campbell JB, Cucakovich N. Adjuvanticity of stearyl tyrosine on inactivated poliovirus vaccine. Vaccine 1986; 4:99-104.
45. Nixon-George A, Moran T, Dionne G, Penney CL, Lafleur D, Bona CA. The adjuvant effect of stearyl tyrosine on a recombinant subunit hepatitis B surface antigen. J Immunol 1990; 144:4798-4802.
46. Allison AC, Byars NE, Waters RV. Immunologic adjuvants: Efficacy and safety considerations. In: Nervig PM, Gough PM, Kaeberle ML, Whetstone CA, eds. Advances in Carriers and Adjuvants for Verterinary Biologics. Ames: Iowa State University Press, 1986:91-103.

47. Byars NE, Allison AC. Adjuvant formulation for use in vaccines to elicit both cell-mediated and humoral immunity. Vaccine 1987; 5:223-228.
48. Kenney JS, Hughes BW, Masada MP, Allison AC. Influence of adjuvants on the quantity, affinity, isotype and epitope specificity of murine antibodies. J Immunol Meth 1989; 121:157-166.
49. Allison AC, Byars NE. The development of an adjuvant formulation that elicits cell-mediated and humoral immune responses to virus subunit and other antigens. In: Majde JA, ed. Progress in Leucocyte Biology: Immunopharmacology of Infectious Diseases. New York: Alan R Liss, 1987(6):191-201.
50. Allison AC, Byars NE. An adjuvant formulation that selectively elicits the formation of antibodies of protective isotypes and of cell-mediated immunity. J Immunol Meth 1986; 95:157-168.
51. Hunter RL, Bennett B. Modulation of antigen presentation and host mediators by block copolymer adjuvants. In: Majde JA, ed. Progress in Leucocyte Biology: Immunopharmacology of Infectious Diseases. New York: Alan R Liss, 1987:181-190.
52. Schmolka IR. A review of block polymer surfactants. J Am Oil Chem Soc 1977; 54:110-116.
53. Hunter RL, Bennett B. The adjuvant activity of nonionic block polymer surfactants. II. Antibody formation and inflammation related to the structure of triblock and octablock copolymers. J Immunol 1984; 133(6):3167-3175.
54. Zigterman GJWJ, Snippe H, Jansze M, Ernste EBHW, De Reuver MJ, Willers JMN. Nonionic block polymer surfactants enhance immunogenicity of pneumococcal hexasaccharide-protein vaccines. Infect Immunol 1988; 56(5):1391-1393.
55. Zigterman GJWJ, Schotanus K, Ernste EBHW, Van Dam GJ, Jansze M, Snippe H, Willers JMN. Nonionic block polymer surfactants modulate the humoral immune response against *Streptococcus pneumoniae*-derived hexasaccharide-protein conjugates. Infect Immunol 1989; 57(9):2712-2718.
56. Howerton DA, Hunter RL, Ziegler HK, Check IJ. Induction of macrophage Ia expression in vivo by a synthetic block copolymer L81. J Immunol 1990; 144:1578-1584.
57. Litwin SD, Singer JM. The adjuvant action of latex particulate carriers. J Immunol 1965; 95(6):1147-1152.
58. Kreuter J, Speiser PP. New adjuvants on a polymethylmethacrylate base. Infect Immunol 1976; 13(1):204-210.
59. Kreuter J, Mauler R, Gruschkau H, Speiser PP. The use of new polymethylmethacrylate adjuvants for split influenza vaccines. Expl Cell Biol 1976; 44:1219.
60. Kreuter J, Haenzel I. Mode of action of immunological adjuvants: some physicochemical factors influencing the effectivity of polyacrylic adjuvants. Infect Immunol 1978; 19(2):667-675.
61. Kreuter J, Nefzger M, Liehl E, Czok R, Voges R. Distribution and elimination of poly(methyl methacrylate) nanoparticles after subcutaneous administration to rats. J Pharm Sci 1983; 72(10):1146-1149.

62. Kreuter J, Berg U, Liehl E, Soliva M, Speiser PP. Influence of the particle size on the adjuvant effect of particulate polymeric adjuvants. Vaccine 1986; 4:125-129.

63. Kreuter J, Liehl E, Berg U, Soliva M, Speiser PP. Influence of hydrophobicity on the adjuvant effect of particulate polymeric adjuvants. Vaccine 1988; 6:253-256.

64. Ostroff GR, Easson DD, Jamas S. Vaccine adjuvant applications of novel yeast carbohydrate microcapsules. Abstract. International Conference for Infectious Diseases. July 15-19, 1990.

65. Tam JP. Synthetic peptide vaccine design. Synthesis and properties of a high density multiple antigenic peptide system. Proc Natl Acad Sci USA 1988; 85: 5409-5413.

66. Tam JP, Lu Y-A. Vaccine engineering: chemically unambiguous synthetic peptide vaccine. Abstract. International conference on advances in AIDS vaccine research, Third annual meeting of the national cooperative vaccine development groups for AIDS. October 1-5, 1990.

67. Pearson MN, Raffel S. Macrophage-digested antigen as inducer of delayed hypersensitivity. J Exp Med 1971; 133:494-505.

68. Parish CR. Preferential induction of cell-mediated immunity by chemically modified sheep erythrocytes. Eur J Immunol 1972:143-151.

69. Tom BH. An overview: Liposomes and immunobiology-macrophages, liposomes, and tailored immunity. In: Tom BH and Six HR, eds. Liposomes and Immunobiology. New York: Elsevier-North Holland, 1980:3-22.

70. Turk JL. In: Neuberger A, Tatum EL, eds. Delayed Hypersensitivity. New York: John Wiley, 1967.

71. Coon J, Hunter R. Selective induction of delayed hypersensitivity by a lipid conjugated protein antigen which is localized in thymus dependent lymphoid tissue. J Immunol 1973; 110(1):183-190.

72. Dailey MO, Hunter RL. The role of lipid in the induction of hapten-specific delayed hypersensitivity and contact sensitivity. J Immunol 1974; 112(4): 1526-1534.

73. Prager MD, Baechtel FS, Gordon WC, Mauldin S, Steinberg J, Sanderson A. Effect of dimethyldioctadecylammonium bromide (DDA) on immunologic parameters and anti-tumor responses. In: Tom BH and Six HR, eds. Liposomes and Immunobiology. New York: Elsevier-North Holland, 1980:39-48.

74. Prager MD, Gordon WC. Enhanced response to chemoimmunotherapy and immunoprophylaxis with the use of tumor-associated antigens with a lipophilic agent. Cancer Res 1978; 38:2052-2057.

75. Prager MD, Gordon WC. Immunoprophylaxis and therapy with lipid conjugated lymphoma cells. GANN Mono Cancer Res 1979; 23:143-150.

76. Nicolotti RA, Kinsky SC. Immunogenicity of liposomal model membranes sensitized with mono(p-azobenzenearsonic acid) tyrosylphosphatidylethanolamine derivatives. Antibody formation and delayed hypersensitivity reaction. Biochemistry 1975; 14:2331-2337.

77. Van Houte AJ, Snippe H, Peulen GTM, Willers JMN. Characterization of immunogenic properties of haptened liposomal model membranes in mice. III. Specificity of delayed-type hypersensitivity and antibody formation. Immunol 1981; 42:233-239.

78. Raz A, Bucana C, Fogler WE, Poste G, Fidler IJ. Biochemical, morphological, and ultrastructural studies on the uptake of liposomes by murine macrophages. Cancer Res 1981; 41:487-494.

79. Coon J, Hunter R. Properties of conjugated protein immunogens which selectively stimulate delayed-type hypersensitivity. J Immunol 1975; 114(5): 1518-1522.

80. Dailey MO, Hunter RL. Induction of cell-mediated immunity to chemically modified antigens in guinea pigs. I. Characterization of the immune response to lipid-conjugated protein antigens. J Immunol 1977; 118(3):957-962.

81. Janeway CA Jr, Horowitz M, Dailey MO, Hunter RL, Wigzell H. Lipid-modified antigens. I. Specificity of guinea pig T lymphocyte responses and I-region restriction. J Immunol 1979; 122(4):1482-1488.

82. Dailey MO, Post W, Hunter RL. Induction of cell-mediated immunity to chemically modified antigens in guinea pigs. II. The interaction between lipid-conjugated antigens, macrophages, and T lymphocytes. J Immunol 1977; 118(3):963-970.

83. Migliore-Samour D, Floc'h F, Maral R, Werner GH, Jolles P. Adjuvant activities of chemically modified water-soluble substances from *Mycobacterium tuberculosis*. Immunol 1977; 33:477-484.

84. Parant MA, Audibert FM, Chedid LA, Level MR, Lefrancier PL, Choay JP, Lederer E. Immunostimulalant activities of a lipophilic muramyl dipeptide derivative and of desmuramyl peptidolipid analogs. Infect Immunol 1980; 27(3):826-831.

85. Jolivet M, Sache E, Audibert F. Biological studies of lipophilic MDP-derivatives incorporated in liposomes. Immunol Commun 1981; 10(6):511-522.

86. Migliore-Samour D, Bouchaudon J, Floc'h F, Zerial A, Ninet L, Werner GH, Jolles P. A short lipopeptide, representative of a new family of immunological adjuvants devoid of sugar. Life Sciences 1980; 26(11):883-888.

87. Floc'h F, Bouchaudon J, Fizames C, Zerial A, Dutruc-Rosset G, Werner GH. Lauroyltetrapeptide (RP-40639) and related lipopeptides: A novel class of synthetic immunomodulating agents. Correlates in Pharmacostructures: Drugs of the Future 1984; 9:773-776.

88. Floc'h F, Poirier J. Immunopotentiating activities of a low molecular weight lipopeptide, Rp 56 142—Studies in infectious models. Int J Immunopharmacol 1988; 10(7):863-873.

89. Parish CR. The relationship between humoral and cell-mediated immunity. Transplant Rev 1972; 13:35-66.

90. Jenkins MK, Burrell E, Ashwell JD. Antigen presentation by resting B cells. Effectiveness at inducing T cell proliferation is determined by costimulatory signals, not T cell receptor occupancy. J Immunol 1990; 144(5):1588-1599.

91. Unanue ER, Allen PM. The basis for the immunoregulatory role of macrophages and other accessory cells. Science 1987; 236:551-557.

92. Unanue ER, Cerottini J-C. Antigen presentation. FASEB J 1989; 3:2496-2502.

93. Chestnut RW, Colon S, Grey H. Antigen presentation by normal B cells, B cell tumors, and macrophages: functional and biochemical comparison. J Immunol 1982; 128:1764-1768.

94. Ashwell J, DeFranco A, Paul W, Schwartz R. Antigen presentation by resting B cells: radiosensitivity of the antigen-presentation function and two distinct pathways of T cell activation. J Exp Med 1984; 159:881-905.

95. Roska AD, Lipsky PE. Dissection of the functions of antigen-presenting cells in the induction of T cell activation. J Immunol 1985; 135:2953-2961.

96. Krieger J, Jenis DM, Chestnut RW, Grey H. Studies on the capacity of intact cells and purified Ia from different B cell sources to function in antigen presentation to T cells. J Immunol 1988; 140:388-394.

97. Engelhard VH, Guild BC, Helenius A, Terhorst C, Strominger JL. Reconstitution of purified detergent-soluble HLA-A and HLA-B antigens into phospholipid vesicles. Proc Natl Acad Sci USA 1978; 75(7):3230-3234.

98. Engelhard VH, Strominger JL, Mescher M, Burakoff S. Induction of secondary cytotoxic T lymphocytes by purified HLA-A and HLA-B antigens reconstituted into phospholipid vesicles. Proc Natl Acad Sci USA 1978; 75(11):5688-5691.

99. Lewis JT, McConnell HM. Model lipid bilayer membranes as targets for antibody-dependent, cellular- and complement-mediated immune attack. Ann NY Acad Sci 1978; 308:124-138.

100. Littman DR, Cullen SE, Schwartz BD. Insertion of Ia and H-2 alloantigens into model membranes. Proc Natl Acad Sci USA 1979; 76(2):902-906.

101. Burakoff SJ, Engelhard VH, Kaufman J, Strominger JL. Induction of secondary cytotoxic T lymphocytes by liposomes containing HLA-DR antigens. Nature 1980; 283:495-497.

102. Watts TH, Gariepy J, Schoolnik GK, McConnel HM. T-cell activation by peptide antigen: Effect of peptide sequence and method of antigen presentation. Proc Natl Acad Sci USA 1985; 82:5480-5484.

103. Quill H, Carlson L, Fox BS, Weinstein JN, Schwartz RH. Optimization of antigen presentation to T cell hybridomas by purified Ia molecules in planar membranes. Ia molecule polymorphism determines the antigenic fine specificity of the response to cytochrome c peptides. J Immunol Meth 1987; 98:29-41.

104. Roof RW, Luescher IF, Unanue ER. Phospholipids enhance the binding of peptides to class II major histocompatibility molecules. Proc Natl Acad Sci USA 1990; 87:1735-1739.

105. Wiesmuller K-H, Jung G, Hess G. Novel low-molecular-weight synthetic vaccine against foot-and-mouth disease containing a potent B-cell and macrophage activator. Vaccine 1989; 7:29-33.

106. Wiesmuller K-H, Hess G, Bessler WG, Jung G. Diastereomers of tripal-mitoyl-S-glyceryl-L-cysteinyl carrier adjuvant systems induce different mitogenic and protective immune response. In: Frank F, Testa B, eds. Chirality and Biological Activity. New York: Alan R Liss, 1990:267-272.

107. Deres K, Schild H, Wiesmuller K-H, Jung G, Rammensee H-G. In vivo priming of virus-specific cytotoxic T lymphocytes with synthetic lipopeptide vaccine. Nature 1989; 342:561-564.

108. Braun V. Covalent lipoprotein from the outer membrane of *Escherichia coli*. Biochimica et Biophysica Acta 1975; 415:335-377.

109. Wu HC, Tokunaga M, Tokunaga H, Hayashi S, Giam C-Z. Posttranslational modification and processing of membrane lipoproteins in bacteria. J Cell Biochem 1983; 22:161-171.

110. Resch K, Bessler W. Activation of lymphocyte populations with concanavalin A or with lipoprotein and lipopeptide from the outer cell wall of *Escherichia coli*: Correlation of early membrane changes with induction of macromolecular synthesis. Eur J Biochem 1981; 115:247-252.

111. Bessler WG, Cox M, Lex A, Suhr B, Wiesmuller K-H, Jung G. Synthetic lipopeptide analogs of bacterial lipoprotein are potent polyclonal activators for murine B lymphocytes. J Immunol 1985; 135(3):1900-1905.

112. Wiesmuller K-H, Bessler W, Jung G. Synthesis of the mitogenic S-[2,3-Bis(palmitoyloxy)propyl]-N-palmitoylpentapeptide from *Escherichia coli* lipoprotein. Hoppe-Seyler's Z Physiol Chem 1983; 364:593-606.

113. Chou PY, Fasman GD. Prediction of the secondary structure of proteins from their amino acid sequence. In: Meister A, ed. Advances in Enzymology. Vol. 47. New York: John Wiley, 1978:45-148.

114. Mergler M, Tanner R, Gosteli J, Grogg P. Peptide synthesis by a combination of solid phase and solution methods. I. A new very acid-labile anchor group for the solid phase synthesis of fully protected fragments. Tetrahedron Lett 1988; 29:4005-4008.

115. Bessler WG, Cox M, Wiesmuller KH, Jung G. The mitogenic principle of *Escherichia coli* lipoprotein: B-lymphocyte mitogenicity of the synthetic analogue palmitoyl-tetrapeptide (PAM-SER-SER-ASN-ALA). Biochem Biophys Res Commun 1984; 121(1):55-61.

116. Bessler WG, Johnson RB, Wiesmuller KH, Jung G. B-lymphocyte mitogenicity in vitro of a synthetic lipopeptide fragment derived from bacterial lipoprotein. Hoppe-Seyler's Z Physiol Chem 1982; 363:767-770.

117. Jung G, Becker G, Metzger J, Wiesmuller KH, Bessler WG, Biesert L, Buhring HJ, Muller C. Potent B-lymphocyte mitogens as covalently bound carriers for the presentation of antigens and enhancement of immune response. In: Voelter W, Bayer E, Ovchinnokov YA, Ivanov VT, eds. Chemistry of Peptides and Proteins. Vol. 3. Proceedings of the Fifth USSR-FRG Symposium on Chemistry of Peptides and Proteins. Odessa, USSR, May 16-20, 1985:351-362.

118. Bessler WG, Wiesmuller K, Scheuer W, Johnson RB. Synthetic peptide membranes. In: Voelter W, Bayer E, Ovchinnikov YA, Wunsch E, eds. Chemistry of Peptides and Proteins. Vol. 2. Proceedings of the Fourth USSR-FRG Symposium on Chemistry of Peptides and Proteins. Tubingen, Federal Republic of Germany, June 8-12, 1982:87-96.

119. Ponsin G, Strong K, Gotto AM Jr, Sparrow JT, Pownall HJ. In vitro binding of synthetic acylated lipid-associating peptides to high-density lipoproteins: Effect of hydrophobicity. Biochemistry 1984; 23:5337-5342.

120. Ono S, Lee S, Mihara H, Aoyagi H, Kato T, Yamasaki N. Design and synthesis of basic peptides having amphipathic b-structure and their interaction with phospholipid membranes. Biochim Biophys Acta 1990; 1022:237-244.

121. Eibl H. An improved method for the preparation of 1,2-isopropylidene-sn-glycerol. Chem Phys Lipids 1981; 28:1-5.

122. Baer E, Fischer HOL. L(+)Propylene glycol. J Am Chem Soc 1948; 70:609-610.

123. Hoffmann P, Heinle S, Schade UF, Loppnow H, Ulmer AJ, Flad H-D, Jung G, Bessler WG. Stimulation of human murine adherent cells by bacterial lipoprotein and synthetic lipopeptide analogues. Immunobiol 1988; 177:158-170.

124. Wolf B, Hauschildt S, Uhl B, Metzger J, Jung G, Bellser WG. Localization of the cell activator lipopeptide in bone marrow-derived macrophages by electron energy loss spectroscopy (EELS). Immunol Lett 1989; 20:121-126.

125. Cambier JC, Ransom JT. Molecular mechanisms of transmembrane signalling in B lymphocytes. In: Paul WE, Fathman CG, Metzger H, eds. Annual Reviews in Immunology. Vol. 5. Palo Alto, CA: Annual Reviews, 1987:175-199.

126. Adams DO. Molecular interactions in macrophage activation. Immunol Today 1989; 10:33-35.

127. Jung G, Wiesmuller K-H, Becker G, Buhring H-J, Bessler WG. Increased production of specific antibodies by presentation of the antigen determinants with covalently coupled lipopeptide mitogens. Angew Chem Int Ed Engl 1985; 24(10):872-873.

128. Lex A, Wiesmuller K-H, Jung G, Bessler WG. A synthetic analogue of *Escherichia coli* lipoprotein, tripalmitoyl pentapeptide, constitutes a potent immune adjuvant. J Immunol 1986; 137(6):2676-2681.

129. Prass W, Ringsdorf H, Bessler W, Wiesmuller K-H, Jung G. Lipopeptides of the N-terminus of *Escherichia coli* lipoprotein: synthesis, mitogenicity and properties in monolayer experiments. Biochim Biophys Acta 1987; 900:116-128.

130. Uemura K-I, Claflin JL, Davie JM, Kinsky SC. Immune response to liposomal model membranes: Restricted IgM and IgG anti-dinitrophenyl antibodies produced in guinea pigs. J Immunol 1975; 114(3):958-961.

131. Tan L, Loyter A, Gregoriadis G. Incorporation of reconstituted influenza virus envelopes into liposomes: Studies of the immune response in mice. Biochem Soc Trans 1989; 17:129-130.

132. Burkhanov SA, Mazhul LA, Torchilin VP, Ageyeva ON, Saatov TS, Andzhanaridze OG. Protective action of influenza-virus surface antigens incorporated in liposomes in various methods of immunization. Viprosy Birusologii 1988; 33(2):151-153.

133. Bruyere T, Wachsmann D, Klein J-P, Scholler M, Frank RM. Local response in rat to liposome-associated *Straptococcus mutans* polysaccharide-protein conjugate. Vaccine 1987; 5:39-42.

134. Thibodeau L, Chagnon M, Flamand L, Oth D, Lachapelle L, Tremblay C, Montagnier L. Role of liposomes in the presentation of HIV envelope glycoprotein and the immune response in mice. CR Acad Sci Paris 1989; 309(20):741-747.

135. Kramp WJ, Six HR, Kasel JA. Postimmunization clearance of liposome entrapped adenovirus type 5 hexon. Proc Soc Exp Bio Med 1982; 169:135-139.

136. Raz A, Bucana C, Fogler WE, Poste G, Fidler IJ. Biochemical, morphological, and ultrastructural studies on the uptake of liposomes by murine macrophages. Cancer Res 1981; 41:487-494.

137. Schroit AJ, Fidler IJ. Effects of liposome structure and lipid composition on the activation of the tumoricidal properties of macrophages by liposomes containing muramyl dipeptide. Cancer Res 1982; 42:161-167.

138. Phillips N, Chedid L. Anti-infectious activity of liposomal muramyl dipeptides in immunodeficient CBA/N mice. Infect Immunol 1987; 55:1426-1430.

139. Sanchez Y, Ionescu-Matiu I, Dreesman GR, Kramp W, Six HR, Hollinger FB, Melnick JL. Humoral and cellular immunity to hepatitis B virus-derived antigens: comparative activity of Freund complete adjuvant, alum and liposomes. Infect Immunol 1980; 30(3):728-733.

140. Kersten GFA, Teerlink T, Derks HJGM, Verkleij AJ, Van Wezel TL, Crommelin DJA, Beuvery EC. Incorporation of the major outer membrane protein of *Neisseria gonorrhoeae* in saponin-lipid complexes (ISCOMs): Chemical analysis, some structural features, and comparison of their immunogenicity with three other antigen delivery systems. Infect Immunol 1988; 56:432-438.

141. McWilliam AS, Stewart GA. Production of multilamellar, small unilamellar and reverse-phase liposomes containing house dust mite allergens. J Immunol Meth 1989; 121:53-69.

142. Szoka F, Papahadjopoulos D. Comparative properties and methods of preparation of liposomes. Ann Rev Biophys Bioeng 1980; 9:467-508.

143. Therien H-M, Shahum E. Importance of physical association between antigen and liposomes in liposomes adjuvanticity. Immunol Lett 1989; 22:253-258.

144. Eichler HG, Senior J, Stadler A, Pfundner P, Gregoriadis G. Kinetics and disposition of fluorescein-labelled liposomes in healthy human subjects. Eur J Clin Pharmacol 1988; 34:475-479.

145. Alving CR, Richards RL, Egan JE, Schultz C, Gordon DM, Fries LF. Liposomes containing lipid A: A potent nontoxic adjuvant for a human malaria sporozoite vaccine. Abstract. International conference on advances in AIDS vaccine research, Third annual meeting of the national cooperative vaccine development groups for AIDS. October 1-5, 1990.

146. Martin FJ, Papahadjopoulos D. Irreversible coupling of immunoglobulin fragments to preformed vesicles. J Biol Chem 1982; 257:286-288.

147. Shen D-F, Huang A, Huang L. An improved method for covalent attachment of antibody to liposomes. Biochim Biophys Acta 1982; 689:31-37.

148. Huang A, Yusao YS, Kennel SJ, Huang L. Characterization of antibody covalently coupled to liposomes. Biochim Biophys Acta 1982; 716:140-150.

149. Leserman LD, Machy P, Barbet J. Covalent coupling of monoclonal antibodies and protein A to liposomes: Specific interaction with cells in vitro and in vivo. In: Gregoriadis G, ed. Liposome Technology. Vol. III. Boca Raton: CRC Press, 1983:29-40.

150. Derksen JTP, Scherphof GL. An improved method for the covalent coupling of proteins to liposomes. Biochim Biophys Acta 1985; 814:151-155.

151. Chua M-M, Fan S-T, Karush F. Attachment of immunoglobulin to liposomal membrane via protein carbohydrate. Biochim Biophys Acta 1984; 800:291-300.

152. Bogdanov AA Jr, Klibanov AL, Torchilin VP. Protein immobilization on the surface of liposomes via carbodiimide activation in the presence of N-hydroxysulfosuccinimide. Eur Biochem Soc 1988; 231(2):381-384.

153. Torchilin VP, Goldmacher VS, Smirnov VN. Covalent studies on covalent and noncovalent immobilization of protein molecules on the surface of liposomes. Biochem Biophys Res Comm 1978; 85(3):983-990.

154. Van Rooijen N, Van Nieuwmegen R. Liposomes in immunology: Evidence that their adjuvant effect results from surface exposition of the antigen. Cell Immunol 1980; 49:402-407.

155. Heath et al., U.S. Patent 4,565,696, January 21, 1986.

156. Gregoriadis G, Davis D, Davies A. Liposomes as immunological adjuvants: antigen incorporation studies. Vaccine 1987; 5:145-151.

157. Shahum E, Therien H-M. Comparative effect on humoral response of four different proteins covalently linked on BSA-containing liposomes. Cellular Immunol 1989; 123:36-43.

158. Dal Monte PR, Szoka FC. Antigen presentation by B cells and macrophages of cytochrome c and its antigenic fragment when conjugated to the surface of liposomes. Vaccine 1989; 7:401-408.

159. Weissig V, Lasch J, Gregoriadis G. Covalent coupling of sugars to liposomes. Biochim Biophys Acta 1989; 1003:54-57.

160. Brynestad K, Babbit B, Huang L, Rouse BT. Liposomal peptide as a subunit vaccine. In: Marshak D, Liu D, eds. Therapeutic Peptides and Proteins: Formation, Delivery and Targeting. Cold Spring Harbor, NY: Cold Spring Harbor Laboratories, 1989:99-105.

161. Brynestad K, Babbit B, Huang L, Rouse BT. Influence of peptide acylation, liposome incorporation and synthetic immunomodulators on the immunogenicity of peptides corresponding to glycoprotein D of herpes simplex virus: Implications for subunit vaccines. Abstract. Second annual meeting of the national cooperative vaccine development groups for AIDS. October 15-18, 1989.

162. Brynestad K, Babbitt B, Huang L, Rouse BT. Influence of peptide acylation, liposome incorporation, and synthetic immunomodulators on the immunogenicity of a 1-23 peptide of glycoprotein D of herpes simplex virus: Implications for subunit vaccines. J Virol 1990; 64(2):680-685.

163. Goodman-Snitkoff G, Heimer EP, Danho W, Felix AM, Mannino RJ. Induction of antibody production to synthetic peptides via peptide-phospholipid complexes. In: Technological Advances in Vaccine Development. New York: Alan R Liss, 1988:335-344.

164. Goodman-Snitkoff G, Eisele LE, Mannino RJ. The immune response to peptide-phospholipid conjugates. Abstract. Second annual meeting of the national cooperative vaccine development groups for AIDS. October 15-18, 1989.

165. Mannino RJ, Eisels LE, Goodman-Snitkoff G. Liposomes in the production of subunit vaccines: The immune response to peptide-phospholipid conjugates. Abstract. Liposome Research Days. February 28-March 2, 1990.

166. Goodman-Snitkoff G, Eisele LE, Heimer EP, Felix AM, Andersen TT, Fuerst TR, Mannino RJ. Defining minimal requirements for antibody production to peptide antigens. Vaccine 1990; 8:257-262.

167. Abbas AK. Cellular interactions in the immune response. The roles of B lymphocytes and interleukin-4. Am J Pathol 1987; 129:25-33.

168. Snapper CM, Paul WE. Interferon-gamma and B cell stimulatory factor-1 reciprocally regulate Ig isotype production. Science 1987; 236:944-947.

169. Vitetta ES, Bossie A, Fernandez-Botran R, Myers CD, Oliver KG, Sanders VM, Stevens TL. Interaction and activation of antigen-specific T and B cells. Immunol Rev 1987; 99:193-239.

170. Dal Monte P, Szoka FC. Effect of liposome encapsulation on antigen presentation in vitro. Comparison of presentation by peritoneal macrophages and B cell tumors. J Immunol 1989; 142:1437-1443.

171. Babbitt BP, Allen PM, Matsueda G, Haber E, Unanue ER. Binding of immunogenic peptides to Ia histocompatibility molecules. Nature 1985; 317:359-361.

172. Buus S, Sette A, Grey HM. The interaction between protein-derived immunogenic peptides and Ia. Immunol Rev 1987; 98:115-141.

173. Etlinger HM, Gillessen D, Lahm H-W, Matile H, Schonfeld H-J, Trzeciak A. Use of prior vaccinations for the development of new vaccines. Reports 1990; 249:423-425.

174. Finberg R, Mescher M, Burakoff SJ. The induction of virus-specific cytotoxic T lymphocytes with solubilized viral and membrane proteins. J Exp Med 1978; 148:1620-1627.

175. Staerz UD, Karasuyama H, Garner AM. Cytotoxic T lymphocytes against a soluble protein. Nature 1987; 329:449-451.

176. Carbone FR, Moore MW, Sheil MM, Bevan MJ. Induction of cytotoxic T lymphocytes by primary in vitro stimulation with peptides. J Exp Med 1988; 167:1767-1779.

177. Moore MW, Carbone FR, Bevan MJ. Introduction of soluble protein into the class I pathway of antigen processing and presentation. Cell 1988; 54: 777-785.

178. Carbone FR, Bevan MJ. Induction of ovalbumin-specific cytotoxic T cells by in vivo peptide immunization. J Exp Med 1989; 169:603-612.

179. Takahashi H, Houghten R, Putney SD, Margulies DH, Moss B, Germain RN, Berzofsky JA. Structural requirements for class I MHC molecule-mediated antigen presentation and cytotoxic T cell recognition of an immunodominant determinant of the human immunodeficiency virus envelope protein. J Exp Med 1989; 170:2023-2035.

2

HIV-1 Virus-Like Particles as a Source of Antigen for AIDS Vaccines

Anna Aldovini and Richard A. Young

*Whitehead Institute for Biomedical Research
and Massachusetts Institute of Technology
Cambridge, Massachusetts*

HIV-1 VIRUS-LIKE PARTICLES

Several strategies permit the production of particles that contain some or most components of the human immunodeficiency virus type 1 (HIV-1). There are two general types of particle vaccine candidates: noninfectious HIV virions and subunit particles that are composed of single viral proteins. Noninfectious HIV-1 virions can be obtained by introducing specific mutations into the viral genome. Subunit particles are typically generated by producing a viral protein that is capable of assembly into a particle in host cells.

Viruslike particles are a potential source of antigen for HIV vaccine candidates. In this capacity, particles have several attractive features over other sources of HIV antigens. Particles are likely to be safer than live attenuated HIV vaccine candidates. The protein components of particles should retain their conformational integrity better than do their counterparts in viruses killed by heat or chemical treatment. Similarly, the components of particles are more likely to be stable than unassembled recombinant viral proteins. Finally, the purification of particles can be faster and less expensive than the purification of other types of recombinant viral proteins.

NONINFECTIOUS HIV VIRIONS

A variety of HIV mutations have been constructed that cause the production of viruses that appear to be noninfectious or severely attenuated. Among these are mutations that affect packaging of genomic RNA into the virion (1-3) and mutations in the viral protease (4). As vaccine candidates, the major advantage of these apparently noninfectious virions is that they contain almost all the components of the complete virus.

Packaging is the process by which viral proteins and RNA get together to form an infectious particle. Unspliced genomic RNA is an indispensable component of the retrovirus particle, and the packaging process can discriminate between unspliced viral RNA and spliced viral or cellular mRNAs. This discrimination is very likely the result of interaction between specific viral RNA sequences and viral proteins (5,6).

RNA sequences essential for packaging have been mapped to a site near the 5' end of the viral genome in avian and murine retroviruses (7-12). The HIV-1 ψ site is located in the 5' leader region of the genomic viral RNA, and deletions located immediately 3' to the splice donor site as small as 19 base pairs can produce a defect in packaging (1,2). This site occurs within intervening sequences that are removed during splicing, producing an unpackageable RNA. HIV-1 ψ site mutants exhibit normal patterns of gene expression in transfected cells, and the viral particles produced by these mutants, while lacking detectable RNA, appear normal in protein composition (2).

HIV-1 nucleocapsid mutations can also produce an RNA packaging defect (2,3). A zinc finger motif of the form $CysX_2CysX_4HisX_4Cys$ is a common feature of the carboxyl terminus of the gag precursor in all retroviruses (13). As nucleic acid binding properties have been attributed to proteins containing zinc finger motifs (14), a role for the zinc finger in RNA binding has been investigated for the Rous sarcoma (RSV) and the Moloney leukemia (MLV) viruses (15) and for HIV-1 (2,3). In RSV, deletion of the first of the two zinc finger motifs abolishes RNA packaging and infectivity. Deletion of the second motif reduces viral infectivity approximately 100-fold. Both zinc fingers are important for 70S RNA dimer formation (16,17). Similar results have been observed for MLV, where the lack of packaging of genomic RNA seems to correlate with nonspecific packaging of spliced viral RNA and cellular mRNAs (18-20). In HIV-1, amino acid substitutions affecting one or more of the cysteine residues in either of the two zinc-finger motifs in the nucleocapsid protein (NC) p7 produce a viral particle that lacks full-length genomic RNA (2).

Analysis of HIV-1 packaging mutants has revealed that assembly of HIV-1 capsids occurs in the absence of RNA packaging. A particle whose protein composition is similar to that of wild-type virions is assembled even when the genomic RNA cannot be packaged. Mutations in the zinc fingers of p7, a protein that is probably directly involved in RNA packaging, do not affect capsid assembly, indicating that the zinc finger domain of p7 does not play a role in assembly of the protein components of the virus.

HIV-1 packaging mutations reduce viral infectivity at least 10^5-fold (3), but it is not yet clear that these mutants are absolutely noninfectious. Nonetheless, we and others have been unable to detect infectious HIV-1 among particles produced by any of the packaging mutants investigated thus far (2,3). Murine retroviruses can recombine with endogenous retroviral sequences present in the host genome, and murine retroviral packaging mutants revert at significant frequencies via recombination (9,10). Sequences with a similar level of homology to HIV-1 are not found in the human genome, and HIV-1 packaging mutants do not appear to have the opportunity to revert via these homologous recombination mechanisms.

Multiple mutations can be introduced into the HIV-1 genome to produce a packaging mutant virus with a very low probability of being infectious. Potential reversion of point mutations in the nucleocapsid protein can be minimized by altering multiple cysteine residues in the zinc finger motif of the NC p7 (2). In addition, the simultaneous presence of a ψ site deletion mutation would further reduce the possibility of fortuitous packaging. If necessary, the HIV-1 genome containing packaging mutations can be divided into two independent constructs stably integrated in a cell line, and any rescued genome will be highly defective.

Mutations in the viral protease have also been shown to cause the production of HIV-1 particles that appear to be noninfectious. Mutations that alter amino acid residues crucial for protease function abolish proteolytic processing of the capsid precursor protein (4,21). Viruslike particles are produced by these mutant viruses. These particles appear to be larger and somewhat less electron-dense than wild-type virions. The extent to which the protease deficiency reduces HIV-1 infectivity is not yet clear. As with the HIV-1 packaging mutants, it should be possible to determine whether infectivity is abolished by making similar mutations in simian immunodeficiency virus (SIV) and determining whether very large amounts of mutant virus can produce an infection in macaques.

SUBUNIT PARTICLES

Viruslike particles have also been obtained by expressing certain HIV-1 genes in baculovirus- or vaccinia virus-infected cells, or by producing HIV:Ty hybrid proteins in yeast.

The unprocessed HIV-1 gag precursor protein assemblies in 100-200-nm particles budding from the cell surface when expressed by baculovirus recombinants in infected insect cells (22). These particles, which resemble immature budding viruses, are released in the culture medium of host cells. The gag precursor has been thought to play an important role in the formation of viral particles at the plasma membrane (23). In the baculovirus system, the accumulation of viruslike particles depends on the presence of the gag precursor; maturation of gag proteins within the cell resulted in the loss of particles in the culture medium (22). Budding is dependent on myristylation of the N-terminal glycine residue, and this modification is thought to be involved in membrane association of the protein (24,25).

Recombinant vaccinia viruses that simultaneously express the HIV-1 *gag-pol* and *env* genes have been constructed that direct the formation of viruslike particles that are released into the culture medium of infected cells (D. Panicali, personal communication). These particles contain processed gag and pol polypeptides as well as envelope glycoproteins, and appear to have an electron-dense cylindrical core in electron micrographs. The antibody response in rabbits immunized with the vaccinia recombinants could be boosted with purified particles derived from cells infected with the vaccinia recombinant, supporting the idea that these particles may be useful immunogens.

Hybrid particles have been produced that contain portions of HIV-1 env fused to one of the major structural components of a viruslike particle found in yeast (26). The yeast retrotransposon Ty encodes a set of proteins that are assembled into viruslike particles called Ty-VLPs (27, 28). One of these proteins, p1, can alone form Ty-VLPs (29). When a fusion protein was engineered to contain most of p1 and a portion of HIV gp120, hybrid HIV:Ty-VLPs were produced by yeast cells (26). These particles are not found in the culture medium, but can be readily obtained from extracts of the yeast cells. When injected into rabbits in combination with adjuvant, the HIV:Ty VLPs induced antibody responses to HIV determinants in the particles.

PERSPECTIVES

Viruslike particles have several features that make them attractive candidates for acquired immunodeficiency syndrome (AIDS) vaccine antigen, including safety, conformational stability, and relative ease of purification. We believe that noninfectious packaging mutant virions are particularly attractive because they contain all the protein components of the normal virus, lacking only the RNA genome. This type of vaccine candidate is also appealing because it most closely resembles the inactivated whole SIV vaccines that have provided some degree of protection against SIV in macaques (30,31). The packaging mutant virions may be as safe as the chemical or heat-inactivated virus, but may better retain antigenic characteristics useful in the immune response to vaccination.

There are many interesting questions about the process of HIV-1 particle formation that have yet to be thoroughly studied, but that may provide important information for investigators interested in viruslike particles as antigen for vaccines. For example, we lack good information about the process of capsid protein assembly and about RNA that may be present in viruslike particles. In addition, there are a large number of artist's conceptions of the structure of the complete retroviral capsid, interpreted from electron micrographs of the virus, but there is little information available on the actual molecular structure of HIV-1. The results of X-ray crystallographic studies are likely to help resolve this problem. Nonetheless, it would be of interest to better understand the process of capsid assembly. Do the capsid proteins self-assemble in vivo, or does this process require chaperonins? How does the genomic RNA associate with the capsid proteins? Answers to these questions may help in the design of better viruslike particles for vaccine purposes.

ACKNOWLEDGMENTS

This work was supported by Public Health Service Grant AI26463 from the National Institutes of Health, and by a Burroughs Wellcome Scholar Award.

REFERENCES

1. Lever A, Gottlinger H, Haseltine W, Sodrosky J. Identification of a sequence required for efficient packaging of Human Immunodeficiency Virus Type I RNA into virions. J Virol 1989; 63:4085-4087.

2. Aldovini A, Young RA. Mutations of RNA and protein sequences involved in Human Immunodeficiency Virus Type 1 packaging result in production of noninfectious virus. J Virol 1990; 64:1920-1926.

3. Gorelick RJ, Nigida SM Jr, Bess JW Jr, Arthur LO, Henderson LE, Rein A. Noninfectious Human Immunodeficiency Virus Type 1 mutants deficient in genomic RNA. J Virol 1990; 64:3207-3211.

4. Gottlinger HG, Sodoski JG, Haseltine WA. Role of capsid precursor processing and myristoylation in morphogenesis and infectivity of Human Immunodeficiency Virus Type 1. Proc Natl Acad Sci USA 1989; 86:5781-5785.

5. Varmus H. Form and function of retroviral proviruses. Science 1982; 216: 812-820.

6. Weiss R, Teich N, Coffin J, Temin H. RNA Tumor Virus. Cold Spring Harbor, NY: Cold Spring Harbor Laboratories, 1984.

7. Koyama T, Harada F, Kawai S. Characterization of a Rous Sarcoma Virus mutant defective in packaging its own genomic RNA: Biochemical properties of mutant TK15 and mutant induced transformants. J Virol 1984; 51: 154-162.

8. Linial M, Medeiros E, Hayward WS. An avian oncovirus mutant (SE21Q1b) deficient in genomic RNA: biological and biochemical characterization. Cell 1978; 15:1371-1381.

9. Mann R, Mulligan RC, Baltimore D. Construction of a retrovirus packaging mutant and its use to produce helper free defective retrovirus. Cell 1983; 33:153-159.

10. Mann R, Baltimore D. Varying the position of a retrovirus packaging sequence results in the encapsidation of both unspliced and spliced RNAs. J Virol 1985; 54:401-407.

11. Shank PR, Linial M. Avian oncovirus mutant (SE21Q1b) deficient in genomic RNA: characterization of a deletion in the provirus. J Virol 1980; 36:450-456.

12. Watanabe S, Temin HM. Encapsidation sequences for spleen necrosis virus, an avian retrovirus, are between 5' long terminal repeat and the start of *gag* gene. Proc Natl Acad Sci USA 1982; 79:5980-5990.

13. Berg J. Potential metal-binding domains in nucleic acid binding proteins. Science 1986; 232:485-486.

14. Evans RM, Hollenberg SM. Zinc fingers: guilt by association. Cell 1988; 52:1-3.

15. Karpel RL, Henderson LE, Orolszlan S. Interactions of retroviral structural proteins with single-stranded nucleic acids. J Biol Chem 1987; 262:4961-4967.

HIV-1 VIRUS-LIKE PARTICLES AND AIDS VACCINES **49**

16. Meric C, Spahr P-F. Rous sarcoma virus nucleic acid-binding protein p12 is necessary for viral 70S RNA dimer formation and packaging. J Virol 1986; 60:450-459.

17. Meric C, Gouilloud E, Spahr P-F. Mutations in Rous sarcoma virus nucleocapsid protein p12(NC): deletions of cys-his boxes. J Virol 1988; 62:3328-3333.

18. Gorelick RJ, Henderson LE, Hanser JP, Rein A. Point mutants of Moloney murine leukemia virus that fail to package viral RNA: Evidence for specific RNA recognition by a "zinc finger-like" protein sequence. Proc Natl Acad Sci USA 1988; 85:8420-8424.

19. Meric C, Goff SP. Characterization of Moloney murine leukemia virus mutants with single amino-acid substitutions in the cys-his box of the nucleocapsid protein. J Virol 1989; 63:1558-1568.

20. Prats AC, Sarih L, Gabus C, Litvak S, Keith G, Darlix JL. Small finger protein of avain and murine retroviruses has nucleic acid annealing activity and positions the replication primer tRNA onto genomic RNA. J EMBO 1988; 7:1777-1783.

21. Kohl NE, Emini EA, Schleif WA, Davis LJ, Heimbach JC, Dixon RAF, Scolnick EM, Sigal IS. Active human immunodeficiency virus protease is required for viral infectivity. Proc Natl Acad Sci USA 1988; 85:4686-4690.

22. Gheysen D, Jacobs E, de Foresta F, Thiriart C, Francotte M, Thines D, de Wilde M. Assembly and release of HIV-1 precursor Pr55gag virus-like particles from recombinant baculovirus-infected insect cells. Cell 1989; 59:103-112.

23. Stephens EB, Compans RW. Assembly of animal viruses at cellular membranes. Ann Rev Microbiol 1988; 42:489-516.

24. Bryant M, Ratner L. Myristoylation-dependent replication and assembly of human immunodeficiency virus 1. Proc Natl Acad Sci 1990; 87:523-527.

25. Pal R, Reitz MS, Tschachler E, Gallo RC, Sarngadharan MG, Veronese FD. Myristoylation of gag proteins of HIV-1 plays an important role in virus assembly. AIDS Res Hum Retroviruses 1990; 6:721-730.

26. Adams SE, Dawson KM, Gull K, Kingsman SM, Kingsman AJ. The expression of hybrid HIV:Ty virus-like particles in yeast. Nature 1987; 329:68-70.

27. Mellor J, Malim MH, Gull K, Tuite MF, McCready S, Dibbayawan T, Kingsman SM, Kingsman AJ. Reverse transcriptase activity and Ty RNA are associated with virus-like particles in yeast. Nature 1985; 318:583-586.

28. Garfinkel DJ, Boeke JD, Fink GR. Ty element transposition: reverse transcriptase and virus-like particles. Cell 1985; 42:507-517.

29. Adams SE, Mellor J, Gull K, Sim RB, Tuite MF, Kingsman SM, Kingsman AJ. The functions and relationships of Ty-VLP proteins in yeast reflect those of mammalian retroviral proteins. Cell 1987; 49:111-119.

30. Desrosiers RC, Wyand MS, Kodama T, Ringler DJ, Arthur LO, Sehgal PK, Letvin NL, King NW, Daniel D. Vaccine protection against simian im-

munodeficiency virus infection. Proc Natl Acad Sci USA 1989; 86:6353-6357.
31. Murphey-Corb M, Martin LN, Davison-Fairburn B, Montelaro RC, Miller M, West M, Ohkawa S, Baskin GB, Zhang J-Y, Putney SC, Allison AC, Eppstein DA. A formalin-inactivated whole SIV vaccine confers protection in macaques. Science 1989; 246:193-197.

3

Chemically Defined Synthetic Immunogens and Vaccines by the Multiple Antigen Peptide Approach

James P. Tam
Rockefeller University
New York, New York

INTRODUCTION

Among the various strategies used to develop synthetic vaccines, using synthetic peptide is perhaps the most appealing, in both conceptual simplicity and the feasibility of large-scale production (1-3). Synthetic peptide vaccine is a minimalistic approach that uses a few of the epitopic sites on a protein. An epitopic site is usually a small segment of 10 or fewer amino acids. B-cell epitopic (humoral response) or peptide antigenic sites can elicit neutralizing antibodies that confer protection against infection, while the T-cell epitope (cell-mediated immune response) may help to enhance immunogenicity and generate immunological memory. The small size of a peptide antigen makes it accessible to design and synthesis by the present technology of peptide synthesis either on the laboratory scale for animal testing or in large-scale production for clinical trials. In addition, by keeping only the essential epitopes and eliminating all other unwanted portions of the protein or organism, a synthetic peptide vaccine would provide, in theory, the desired properties of selectivity, stability, and safety of an idealized synthetic vaccine. However, the potential of such a vaccine against infectious diseases has yet to be realized. Rather, peptide antigen remains an attractive and valuable tool in the laboratory for the preparation of site-specific antibodies for various biochemical and functional studies (4-8).

Several limitations of the synthetic peptide vaccine contribute to this state of affairs. A major limitation is the use of a protein carrier. Protein carriers are usually large when compared to the peptide antigen. Thus, the peptide antigen represents only a minor fraction of the total molecular weight of the antigen-carrier conjugate. Similarly, the desirable antibodies may represent only a minor fraction of the total amount of antibodies produced. Other possible problems attendant with the use of a protein carrier include the creation of many irrelevant epitopes that cause carrier toxicity (9) and ectopic suppression (10), which are highly undesirable for human vaccines. Another limitation is the chemical ambiguity of the antigen-protein carrier conjugate, which hinders consistent batch-to-batch production of vaccines for humans. However, the most serious problem may be the low immunogenicity induced by the peptide-protein carrier conjugate, partly because the amount of desired antigens being attached to the protein carrier is usually small. Furthermore, the complexity of attaching peptide antigens to large proteins also limits the incorporation of more than one epitope to the protein carrier. The purpose of this chapter is to address some of these limitations and, at the same time, to introduce a new approach to prepare chemically defined synthetic peptide immunogens that may overcome these limitations.

The new approach developed recently in our laboratory (11-24) is referred to as the multiple antigen peptide (MAP) approach. As the name implies, the MAP approach, using a small core matrix comprised of oligomeric lysine, is a unique presentation system of amplifying peptide antigens into multiple copies. As a result, this approach provides a very high density of peptide antigens at the surface and a nonprotein core matrix as a scaffolding that supports the peptide antigens. This approach replaces the conventional approach of using a protein carrier and thus eliminates many of the disadvantages associated with its use.

This chapter is organized into three parts. The first part briefly describes the concept and method of the MAP approach. The second part describes the properties and characteristics expected of it. The final part provides examples of using the MAP approach for the design and preparation of vaccines against hepatitis and malaria.

THE MAP APPROACH: CONCEPT AND METHOD

Conceptual Framework

Since the central problem lies in the undesirability of the protein carrier, the MAP approach is aimed at replacing it with a small structural unit that can amplify peptide antigens without the disadvantages attendant to a protein carrier. Thus, the conceptual framework of the MAP approach is based on the design of a small core matrix with the following properties: 1) nonimmunogenicity, 2) ability to amplify the peptide antigens to a macromolecule, 3) flexibility of incorporating multiple epitopes, and 4) accessibility to design and chemical synthesis. A core matrix consisting of branching trifunctional amino acids such as lysine would satisfy these requirements (11).

Since lysine contains two amino groups, each level (n) of propagation will produce $2^n - 1$ of lysine and 2^n of reactive amino ends. Thus, the first level of the core matrix, consisting of one lysine, contains two amino groups; the second level, consisting of three lysines, contains four amino groups; the third level, consisting of seven lysines, contains eight amino groups, and so on (Figure 1). We have found that the second or third level

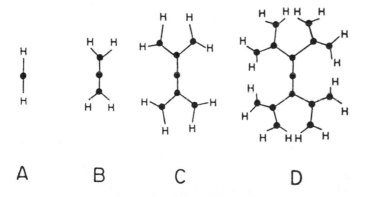

A B C D

Figure 1 Schematic representation of the core matrix of the MAP. (A) First level, divalent; (B) second level, tetravalent; (C) third level, octavalent; and (D) fourth level, hexadecavalent.

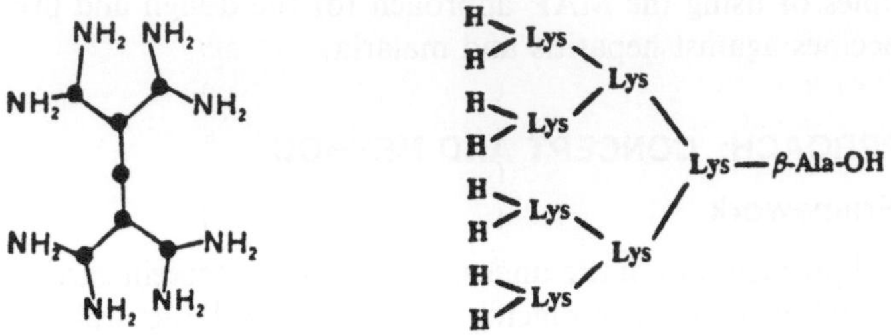

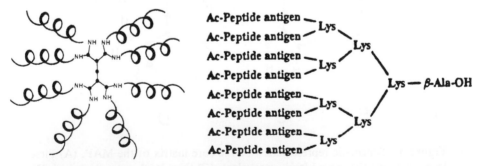

Figure 2   Two schematic representations of the core matrix at the octavalent level.

of propagation is sufficiently suitable for a low-molecular-weight core matrix to replace a high-molecular-weight protein carrier (Figure 2). Peptide antigens are then attached to the amino groups of the lysine scaffolding to give a macromolecule that has a high density of uniformly distributed peptide antigens on the surface (Figure 3). To illustrate this point, a 20-residue peptide derived from the sequence of the foot-and-mouth disease virus (VP1 141-160) attached to an octameric branching core matrix consisting of seven lysines will give a MAP molecule with a MW of about 23,000. The weight percent due to eight copies of peptide antigens accounts for 96%, and the core represented by seven lysines accounts for only 4%. In contrast, the same immunogen when conjugated to a protein carrier such as KLH (MW >1,000,000) will give a low density of peptide antigens randomly distributed on the protein carrier surface.

Figure 3   Two schematic representations of a MAP consisting of the core matrix and peptides.

It is important to emphasize that the key component, the core matrix, is comprised of oligomeric branching rather than polymeric lysine since the core matrix usually consists of either three or seven lysines with a MW of less than 900. Polylysine as a protein carrier is usually a large protein with a MW greater than 100,000 and contains many side-chain cationic groups. In contrast, the core matrix of the oligomeric lysine does not carry any cationic charges since all the side-chain amino groups are coupled as amide bonds to either another lysine or to peptide antigens.

From the practical point of view, the MAP approach to prepare synthetic vaccines has several advantages. First, it can be synthesized de novo in an unambiguous manner. Unlike the conventional peptide-antigen conjugates, the MAP structure can be unequivocally represented by a chemical formula and can be verified with great precision by analytical methods such as amino acid analysis, sequencing, and mass spectrometry. This property is essential for quality control and consistent batch-to-batch production. Second, there is no need for conjugation to a protein carrier that may cause such undesirable immunological reactions as ectopic suppression. Finally, there is the advantage of flexibility that allows the design and engineering of multiple B- and T-cell epitopes. This flexibility is possible due to the sophistication of peptide synthetic methodology to chemically distinguish between the α and ϵ amino groups and its ability of selective attachment of different epitopes of the B- and T-cell origin. The inclusion of T-cell epitopes that could enhance the immunogenicity or elicit cell-mediated immune responses is an important consideration in the design of vaccines. Examples of including T-cell epitopes in the design are given in the "Applications to Vaccines" section later in this chapter. In short, the MAP strategy provides many of the desirable features of the peptide-based vaccine.

Preparation of MAP

For the preparation of MAPs, two general strategies are available: the direct and indirect approaches. The direct approach (11,12) is simpler in execution than the indirect approach (24) since it allows the preparation of the core matrix and the peptide immunogen in a single, continuous operation using the solid-phase peptide synthesis. The indirect approach has the advantage in that purified synthetic peptide fragments are used. The chemistry, which is similar in both approaches, is adopted from the conventional solid-phase peptide methodology (27-29). Both approaches to the preparation of MAPs would be no more complicated than the conventional method for the preparation of monomeric peptide immunogen.

In the direct approach, a peptide antigen and the lysine core are synthesized as a single unit on a resin support (Figure 4). The process begins with a resin support containing a simple amino acid such as glycine, which serves as an internal standard for calculating the molar ratio of other amino acids. The first level of the core matrix contains a diprotected lysine, usually Boc-Lys(Boc) (t-butyloxycarbonyl). Since the protection scheme of the α- and ϵ-amino groups are similar, deblocking the Boc groups followed by coupling a new round of Boc-Lys(Boc) will furnish the next level of the core matrix containing two lysines, one at the α-amino position and the other at the ϵ-amino position. This second level of branching will give a tetrameric MAP containing four amino groups. Similarly, the third-level branching will produce four lysines, eight amino groups, and an octameric MAP. The incorporation of the peptide antigen could begin at either the second level of the tetrameric MAP or the third level of the octameric MAP. In this way, the peptide immunogen is amplified four- or eightfold during the synthesis. At the completion of the synthesis, the peptide immunogen is usually capped with an acetyl group. The necessity for acetylation depends on the origin of the peptide in the protein sequence. Capping is appropriate for peptide derived from the internal sequences since it would remove the charged amino group. The whole unit is then cleaved from the resin support by a strong acid. The product may be purified by dialysis or the usual chromatographic techniques, such

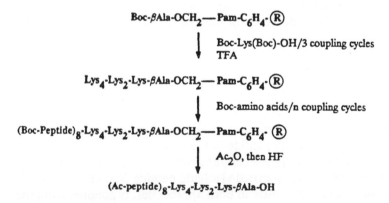

Figure 4   A direct strategy in the synthesis of a MAP by the stepwise solid-phase method.

as gel permeation chromatography, and could be used directly for immunization.

In the indirect approach, the core matrix and the peptide antigens are prepared and purified separately (24). Both components are then recombined to form the MAP-peptide antigen. An advantage of this approach is that a free and purified peptide can be used. Another advantage is that the orientation of the peptide antigen can be arranged as in the native molecule. Thus, this strategy of preparation is particularly suitable for peptide antigens derived from the carboxyl terminus of a protein since the resulting peptide antigen could mimic its native structure, which contains a free and mobile carboxyl end.

A scheme of the indirect approach (Figure 5) utilizes a purified peptide fragment containing a cysteine residue at the amino or carboxyl terminus to react with a core matrix containing chloroacetyl groups. Thiol alkylation of the chloroacetyl group at neutral to slightly alkaline pH combines both components to form a MAP construct with the desired peptide antigen. The preparation of the core matrix terminating with the chloracetyl groups can be conveniently prepared by the solid-phase method using the Boc or Fmoc (fluorenylmethoxycarbonyl) chemistry on a resin support (27-29). Peptide resin containing the oligomeric branching lysine with four or eight amino groups is coupled with chloroacetic acid to form the core matrix containing chloroacetyl moieties. This chloroacetylated core matrix is cleaved by acid (29) from the resin support, and the crude product is usually sufficiently pure for further use.

In a separate synthesis, the desired peptide immunogen is prepared and purified to homogeneity. Purified synthetic peptide fragment containing a cysteine at the amino or carboxyl terminus is ideally suited for conjugation to the chloroacetyl groups of the core matrix (30,31). Thiol alkylation to assemble both components to form a MAP is similar to the conventional conjugation of a peptide antigen to a protein carrier. However, there are two major differences. First, unlike the protein carrier, the molecular weight of the chloroacetylated core matrix is low, less than 2000. Second, each addition of a peptide antigen to the core matrix produces a relatively large increase in molecular weight. These two factors favor the completion of the reaction of the peptide antigen to the core matrix and the resolution of the incomplete reaction products by gel permeation chromatography.

The indirect approach, using purified core matrix and peptide antigen, is similar in concept and practice to the conventional approach for conjugating synthetic peptide to a protein carrier (32-38). Thus, many

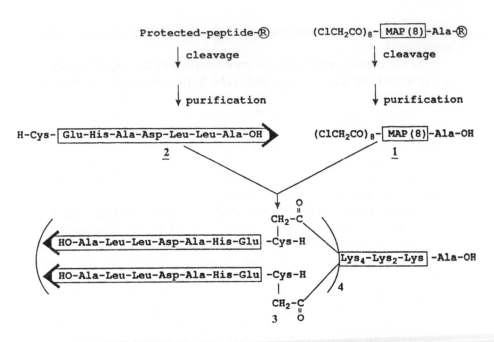

Figure 5   An indirect strategy in the synthesis of a MAP by combining both purified fragments: the chloroacetylated core matrix and a purified peptide containing a cysteine at either the amino or carboxyl terminus. The direction of the arrow indicates the orientation of the peptide from carboxy to amino. The carboxyl terminal octapeptide of human TGFα is used as an example; note that the orientation of the peptide immunogen mimics the native protein with the carboxyl end being free and flexible.

methodological variations of the indirect approach can be envisioned. The described method of using a peptide containing a thiol moiety linked to a chloroacetylated core matrix is only one such variation. Extensions of this method include the use of another haloacetylated core matrix, for example, bromoacetylated or iodoacetylated core matrix. Iodoacetylated core matrix is known to be more reactive toward the thiol alkylation reactions. However, chloroacetylated derivatives would be more stable than the other haloacetylated derivatives in the peptide synthesis steps, such as the HF cleavage step. Similarly, one can envision the use of other heterofunctional cross-linking reagents such as m-maleimidobenzoyl-N-hydroxylsuccinimide ester (MBS) (35), succininimidy 4-(N-maleimidomethyl)cyclohexane-1-carboxylate (SMCC) (36), succinimidyl 4-(p-maleimidophe-nyl)butyrate (SMPD) (37), and N-succinimidyl-3-(2-pyridyldithio)propio-nate (SPDP) (38). Whatever the reagent being used, the indirect approach would provide an advantage of producing a chemically defined peptide immunogen.

Importance of Orientation

The amino and carboxyl fragments of a protein are often the most flexible part of a protein and have been known to be excellent sites for selection as peptide immunogens. The amino fragment of a protein is often variable in the same family of proteins and is suitable to prepare antibodies specific for a particular protein. On the other hand, the COOH peptides are often conserved and not processed in proteins (7), and such fragments may be useful for the preparation of antibodies that could cross-react with homologous proteins of the same family. However, because of the terminal charge (either NH_3^+ or COO^-) and the flexibility of these fragments, the attachment of such peptide fragments to the core matrix by either the amino or carboxyl end could greatly affect the specificity of immune responses.

The importance of the correct orientation of a peptide immunogen attached to a protein carrier has been examined in other peptide-protein conjugates (39). In general, the orientation of the peptide immunogen should mimic the protein structure, which would also govern the orientation of the peptide antigen attached to the core matrix by the MAP approach. For peptide immunogens that are derived from the amino terminal fragments or the internal positions of protein molecules, the direct approach of linking the carboxyl end of these fragments to the core matrix would provide the best results. In such cases, the flexible end of a peptide immunogen would be at the amino terminus. For peptide immunogens that are carboxyl fragments of protein molecules, the direct approach would give an incorrect orientation because the free and flexible carboxyl end is attached to the core matrix. The indirect approach of preparation would overcome this deficiency. By positioning a cysteine residue at the NH_2 terminus of a peptide, the peptide antigen can be attached to the chloroacetylated lysine core matrix at its NH_2 end to give the correct orientation.

The correct orientation has a direct relationship to the antigenicity of the peptide immunogen, as shown in the model system (24) using an eight-residue peptide immunogen of the carboxyl terminal fragment of human transforming growth factor α (TGFα) (40). Conjugation to the core matrix at the amino end of the peptide would give more flexibility of the distal carboxyl end (i.e., residues 46 to 50) than the proximal amino end linked directly to the core matrix. Such an orientation would also resemble the folded and native structure of TGFα. Indeed, antipeptide antisera recognized both the peptide immunogen and TGFα, the protein molecule from which it is derived (Figure 6A). However, the antipeptide failed to recognize the "reverse-immunogen" MAP model even though the same sequence was present, but was attached to the core matrix at a

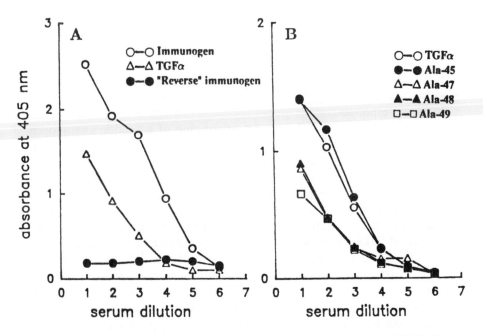

Figure 6 (A) Specificity of antisera and importance of orientation. ELISA immunoreactivity of antisera from a MAP peptide derived from the carboxyl terminus of TGFα, MAP-CEHADLLA. Microtiter wells were coated with (○——○) immunogen, (△——△) TGFα, (●——●) "reverse" immunogen (CEHADLLA-MAP). (B) Determination of antigenic site. Microtiter wells were coated with (○——○) TGFα, (●——●) Ala[45], (△——△) Ala[47], (▲——▲) Ala[48], (□——□) Ala[49] as antigen. Serum dilutions: 1 = 1/16; 2 = 1/64; 3 = 1/256; 4 = 1/1024; 5 = 1/4096; 6 = 1/16,384.

reversed orientation or polarity. In such a case, the COOH end of the same peptide sequence was linked covalently onto the core of MAP. The reason for such specificity was that the antigenic site for the antibodies was located at the distal part of the immunogen containing the last four residues (residues 47-50) as well as the free carboxylic group (see the section "Antigenic Sites and Monospecific Antibodies" for further details).

Other Considerations

The following considerations for the selection of the peptide immunogens have been found to be useful in the MAP strategy.

1. The peptide should be relatively hydrophilic. Hydrophilic peptides are likely to be located on the surface of the protein and have desirable solubility. Note that soluble peptide immunogens always give soluble MAPs.
2. Although various lengths of peptide immunogens ranging from 5 to 37 amino acids have been used in the MAP approach with successful results, the most suitable length of peptide immunogens is in the range of 10 to 20 residues. The effective length appears to be dependent on the species of animals used for immunization. Outbred animals usually respond better than inbred animals, and rabbits are better responders than mice. Peptides of 15 to 20 residues provide best results if mice are used for immunization, but peptides of 10 to 15 residues have been successful in outbred rabbits and guinea pigs. In general, longer peptides are preferred because part of the peptide immunogen often serves as a T-helper cell antigen to enhance immunogenicity (see "Titers and Specificity" below for examples). All the responses to the MAP models have been found to be T-cell dependent, which indicates that the B-cell epitope also acts as a T-cell epitope. There may be greater success in the outbred animals because the repetoire of T-cell epitopes is large and the responses in inbred mice may be MHC-restricted and require specific T-helper epitopes (see the section on malaria in "Applications to Vaccines" later in the chapter).
3. Place the desired antigenic site at one end (amino or carboxyl) of the peptide (see "Antigenic Sites and Monospecific Antibodies"), and use the other end as the attachment to the core matrix.
4. Designs for incorporating diepitopes in the MAP models are discussed in "Applications to Vaccines."

CHARACTERISTICS OF IMMUNE RESPONSES

Titers and Specificity

The immunogenicity of MAPs is observable in the antibody titers. Specific antibody responses are generally produced in the immunization of outbred animals such as rabbits with a success rate of about 90% in our laboratory. Usually, titers of end dilutions to 10^4 or higher are obtained after second or third boostings. Antibodies obtained are usually specific in that they react with either the cognate proteins in solution or denatured proteins in immunoblots. The immune responses are usually lower in mice, particularly if they are inbred strains, due to the MHC restriction. If mice are used, it is advisable to use several strains. The differences in immune responses in animals could be seen in the following examples. An octameric MAP with eight copies of a 12-residue peptide consisting of three repeating tetrapeptides of Asn-Ala-Asn-Pro from the circumsporozoite protein of *Plasmodium falciparum* was found to be nonimmunogenic in BALB/c mice but immunogenic in Black A/J mice and rabbits (11). Similarly, a tetrameric MAP with four copies of an 11-residue peptide (RIQRGPGRAFV) from the gp120 protein of HIV-1 (IIIB strain) was found to be nonimmunogenic in BALB/c mice but immunogenic to rabbits. However, immunogenicity in BALB/c mice was found with the extension of this 11-residue peptide to a 17-residue peptide (KSIRIQRGPGRAFVTIG) of the same MAP construct. The immune response of the 17-residue peptide was due to the inclusion of the T-helper epitope.

A special point that needs to be stressed is the high monospecificity produced by the polyclonal and monoclonal antibodies elicited by peptide immunogens with the MAP approach. The monospecificity may be due to the homogeneity of the peptide immunogen inherent to the MAP construction. Such monospecificity is particularly desirable for the identification and occurrence of specific proteins in tissue distribution and immunostaining. An example of antibody production for this purpose (14) is found in the localization and functional studies of the α subunit of the guanine nucleotide-binding regulatory protein G_o (α_o). Based on the partial sequence obtained from α_o, a polyclonal antibody against this α subunit of the guanine nucleotide-binding protein, G_o, was raised (Asp-Gly-Ile-Ser-Ala-Lys-Asp-Val) by the octameric MAP approach. However, this particular fragment also shares 56 to 66% of sequence homology with several other α subunits (α_i, α_s, and α_T). Antiserum at a final dilution of 1:400 could detect α_o in as little as 0.2 μg of G_o on immunoblots, and at a final dilution of 1:20,000 could detect α_o in 1 μg of G_o on immunoblots

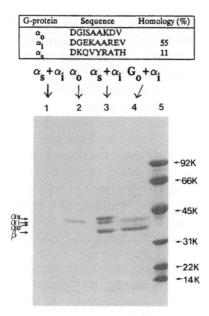

G-protein	Sequence	Homology (%)
α_o	DGISAAKDV	
α_i	DGEKAAREV	55
α_s	DKQVYRATH	11

Figure 7 Specificity of antisera from a MAP peptide (DGISAADV). Left panel shows the immunoblot and the right panel shows the protein by Coomassie staining.

(Figure 7). Antiserum and affinity-purified antibody were specific to α_o. Furthermore, no cross-reactivity was detected in the α subunits of the stimulatory or inhibitory guanine nucleotide-binding regulatory proteins or transducin. The antiserum was then used for immunoblot to locate the distribution of α_o in tissues and allowed detailed immunocytochemical studies to show the tissue distributions and developmental appearance of α_o.

Antigenic Sites and Monospecific Antibodies

A question central to the preparation of peptide immunogens by the MAP approach is the understanding of the molecular basis for the immunogenicity of peptide attached to the core matrix, particularly the location of the dominant antigenic site of a peptide immunogen that binds to the antibodies induced by the MAP constructs. Here, the unique design of the MAP approach makes is possible to provide a clear solution to this question. We have mapped the antigenic sites of many antisera elicited by the MAP models. A general conclusion based on MAPs consisting of peptide immunogens with 20 or fewer residues is that the dominant antigenic site is located on the flexible end, farthest from the core matrix. Furthermore, antigenicity decreases as it traverses from the distal to the proximal end, the least flexible end of the core matrix. Three examples are used below to support the generality of this conclusion.

In the first example (16), a 14-residue peptide immunogen derived from the human T-cell antigen receptor β-chain constant region was used in an octameric MAP construct and elicited highly immunogenic polyclonal and monoclonal antibodies in mice and rabbits. Nearly all these antibodies reacted with the peptide immunogen in its monomeric as well as its octameric form. Moreover, these antibodies also reacted with the intact β-chain protein. To assess the antigenic site, a series of progressively shortened MAPs at the amino terminus was prepared (Figure 8). While 28 of 28 MAbs reacted with the full-length 14-residue MAP, six of 28 MAbs reacted with the 11-residue MAP with the first three amino terminal residues deleted and one of 28 MAbs reacted with the seven-residue MAP with the first seven amino terminal residues deleted. Similarly, polyclonal antisera reacted less strongly with the 11-residue MAP

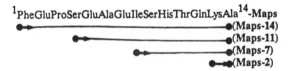

^{1}PheGluProSerGluAlaGluIleSerHisThrGlnLysAla^{14}-Maps

		Recognition by (ELISA)		
Peptide	Size (aa)	MAb	PAb	Control
Maps	14	22/22	+	-
	11	4/22	+/-	-
	7	1/22	-	-
	2	0/22	-	-
Monomeric	14	15/22	+	-
	11	6/22	+/-	-
Polylysine	14	1/22	-	-

Figure 8 Antigenic site of polyclonal (PAb) and monoclonal (MAb) antibodies derived from a 14-residue peptide. The negative control is a mean of 12 values obtained from six different MAbs with irrelevant specificity. The entry on polylysine is derived from the monomeric peptide coupled by water-soluble carbodiimide to polylysine.

and not at all with the seven-residue MAP and lysine core matrix. No antibodies were found to react with the lysine core of the MAP construct. The combined results demonstrate that the amino residues representing the distal end of the 14-residue octameric MAP, which are most exposed and flexible, constitute the antigenic site recognized by the antibodies in the polyclonal sera and by the monoclonal antibodies.

In the second example (24), an eight-residue fragment (residue 43-50, Cys-Glu-His-Ala-Asp-Leu-Leu-Ala-OH) from the carboxyl terminus of human TGFα was used as the immunogen in an octameric MAP construct. Antisera from this MAP reacted with the immunogen, either the monomeric or the octameric MAP form, as well as TGFα. The antisera were used to map the antigenic site of the immunogen by two series of point-substituted analogs of TGFα (Figure 6B) (9). The first series contained an alanine replacement (Figure 6B) while the second contained the corresponding D-amino acid replacement (Figure 9). Both series were intended to complement each other on the importance of the side chain and the conformation of the antigenic region. These analogs were refolded with three disulfide bonds that resembled the native TGFα. Furthermore, they were biologically active in various functional assays. The single Ala-substituted TGFα was intended to show the contribution of side chains to the antigenic site. Diminished reactivity in ELISA to the antisera was observed in analogs Ala-49, Ala-48, and Ala-47. Full activity was restored in analog Ala-45. These results show that amino acids at positions 47 to 49 are important for antigenicity, but information regarding amino acids at positions 50 and 46 could not be obtained because Ala occupies these two positions in the native sequence. To obtain a complete picture, a second series of point-substituted analogs containing replacements with the corresponding D-amino acid was used. Replacement of D-amino acid would disrupt the backbone conformation and show its contribution to antigenicity. Antisera failed to recognize those analogs that contain a single-point substitution at positions 47-50 (analogs D-Ala 50, D-Leu 49, D-Leu 48, and D-Asp 47), but immunoreactivity was restored in analogs that contain a point substitution after position 46, such as D-Ala 46, D-His 45, and D-Glu 44 (Figure 9). These results substantiate those obtained from the Ala series of analogs and show that the antigenicity region is limited to the distal four residues of TGFα. An interesting observation is that the antigenic site is much more sensitive to conformational change because replacement of D-amino acid at any amino acid occupying the terminal positions 47-50 of TGFα completely abolishes immunoreactivity while similar replacement by Ala only diminishes immunoreactivity.

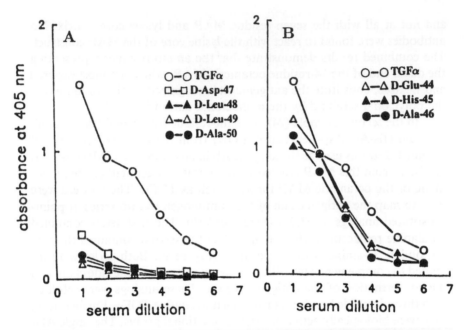

Figure 9   Antigenic sites determined by point-substituted TGFα analogs. ELISA immunoreactivity of antisera derived from an octapeptide-MAP after second immunization. (A) Microtiter wells were coated with (○——○) TGFα, (□——□) D-Asp⁴⁷, (▲——▲) D-Leu⁴⁸, (△——△) D-Leu⁴⁹, (●——●) D-Ala⁵⁰ as antigen. (B) Microtiter wells were coated with (○——○) TGFα, (△——△) D-Glu⁴⁴, (▲——▲) D-His⁴⁵, (●——●) D-Ala⁴⁶ as antigen. Serum dilutions: 1 = 1/16; 2 = 1/64; 3 = 1/256; 4 = 1/1024; 5 = 1/4096; 6 = 1/16,384.

In the third example (22), the antigenic site is determined by the PEPSCAN approach, in which the entire antigenic sequence is "windowed" with the use of a series of overlapping synthetic peptides differing by one amino acid. The PEPSCAN method has a distinct advantage of convenience because synthetic peptides are synthesized on polyethylene rods that are assembled into a molded polyethylene holder designed for 96 rods in the format and spacing of a microtiter plate. This particular format is well suited for the ELISA reactions to study the immune responses of the antiserum, the rod-coupled peptides, and the conjugated solutions in polystyrene microtiter plates.

A 20-residue peptide immunogen of the neutralization epitope of the coat protein (VP1 141-160) of the foot-and-mouth disease virus (FMDV) was incorporated in the octameric MAP format. The MAP approach was compared with those peptide-carrier conjugates of the conventional approach in which VP1(141-160)-Cys was coupled by MBS or by glutaldehyde (GDA) to keyhole limpet hemocyanin (KLH). Two rabbits were inoculated with each immunogen. The MAP constructs induced a very high antipeptide response 8 weeks after immunization (10^4-fold dilution), while the peptides conjugated with KLH induced a lower response. However, neutralization titers of all antisera were similar. The antigenic sites of these antisera were then determined by the PEPSCAN method using overlapping eight-residue synthetic peptides from the region 134-165 of VP1 of FMDV type O (Figure 10). The results revealed that a large population of antibodies raised against MAP were specific to the flexible amino terminal amino acids, and that both rabbits gave a similar response (Figure 10a, b). In contrast, antibodies raised against the peptides conjugated with KLH reacted with different sequences, and each rabbit gave a different response (Figure 10c, d, e, and f). Thus, two conclusions can be drawn from this example. First, these results confirm those two previous examples that the distal and flexible end of the MAP construct is the most

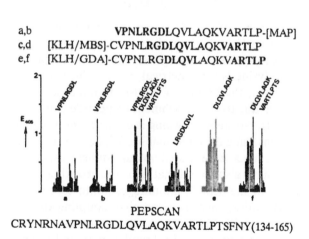

a,b   VPNLRGDLQVLAQKVARTLP-[MAP]
c,d   [KLH/MBS]-CVPNLRGDLQVLAQKVARTLP
e,f   [KLH/GDA]-CVPNLRGDLQVLAQKVARTLP

PEPSCAN
CRYNRNAVPNLRGDLQVLAQKVARTLPTSFNY(134-165)

Figure 10 Specificity and antigen sites of antibody responses from foot-and-mouth disease virus (VP1 141-160) using the PEPSCAN approach. Each line represents the ELISA response of an octapeptide starting from residue 134 of VP1. Six rabbits were tested, and six panels (a to f) represent the immune responses of their antisera.

antigenic. In these examples, peptides ranging from eight to 20 residues consistently show that the distal end is the antigenic site. Second, MAP produces a better controlled antipeptide response than that of the conventional peptide-protein carrier conjugates. This result is not unexpected since MAP is small, chemically defined, and homogeneous in contrast to the conventional peptide-protein conjugate, which is likely to be large, chemically ambiguous, and heterogeneous. Thus, the better controlled antipeptide response by the MAP approach is particularly suited for the production of monospecific antibodies for biochemical studies.

In summary, our combined results suggest that for short peptide immunogens (<20 residues) the distal and most flexible part, away from the attachment site to the core matrix, are most likely to be the antigenic sites. However, this conclusion may not be generalized for longer peptide immunogens (>20 residues), which may be folded into more defined structures with the distal ends looped to the carboxyl ends. Nevertheless, a direct and useful strategy to prepare short peptide immunogens could be derived from these results; i.e., using the MAP approach, the desired antigenic site of a short peptide immunogen should be placed on the distal end of the peptide-MAP construct.

Effect of Number of Branches of the MAP Matrix

The optimal number of branches of the MAP matrix depends on several interplaying factors. These include the interchain steric hinderance, the length and conformation of peptide immunogens, and the molecular size of the end product. Since lysine is asymmetrical, with a short α amino arm and a long ϵ amino arm, the branching is also asymmetrical. The interchain steric hinderance due to the attachment of peptide can be examined by molecular models. No steric crowding is observed with branching up to eight dendritic arms using the molecular model. However, MAPs with 16 branches show steric hinderance. Based on our synthetic experience of the past four years, we have also found that no steric crowding is observed during the synthesis of the peptide immunogens onto core matrix with eight branches. Difficulties, such as incomplete coupling of each amino acid on the core matrix with 16 branches, are sometimes incurred. More importantly, immune responses of MAP models with 16 branches have not shown superiority over those with fewer branches in animals. Thus, MAPs with eight branches are preferred over those with 16 branches. Although steric hinderance is not a problem for the two-branch MAP, its immunogenicity is often inferior to that of the four- and eight-branch MAPs consisting of the same peptide immunogen. For this reason, two-branch MAPs are not used. The choice of four or eight branches in the MAP models depends largely on the length and conformation adopted by the peptide immunogen; from our experience, we have the following generalizations.

1. For most peptide immunogens, the length should be between 10 and 20 residues, and a MAP model of four or eight branches is generally suitable. The desired antigenic site should be at the distal and flexible end of the core matrix.

2. For optimal results in peptides with 10 to 15 residues, MAP branching with eight copies is recommended. This recommendation is based largely on the consideration of the molecular size of the MAP construct. The calculated molecular weight of a MAP containing eight copies of an 11-residue peptide would amount to about 10,500, similar to that of a small protein. However, for peptides with 16 to 20 residues, there is no overwhelming experimental evidence that favors MAPs with eight branches over those with four branches.

3. For peptides with more than 21 residues, MAP branching with four copies is recommended. The molecular size of a MAP containing four copies of a peptide antigen with 24 residues is about 11,000. Conformationally, the average number that spans the length of a globular protein is 22-24 amino acids.

Support for these generalizations is based on the following experiments. In the first (13), monomeric, dimeric, tetrameric, and octameric MAPs of a 20-residue FMDV peptide VP1 141-160 were compared (Figure 11). Neutralizing antibodies obtained from guinea pigs inoculated with a 4-μg dose of the tetrameric and octameric MAPs were similar in both primary and secondary responses. In contrast, dimeric MAP induced no primary neutralizing antibody responses at 4-μg doses and significantly lower responses at 20-μg doses. The monomeric peptide was nonimmunogenic at all the doses examined. These results suggest that for a 20-residue peptide, there is no significant advantage of using the four-branch over the eight-branch MAP.

In the second experiment (20), comparisons were made in a series of MAPs containing a 28-residue peptide composed of tandemly connecting B-cell and T-helper cell epitopes from the circumsporozoite (CS) protein of *Plasmodium berghei*. The B epitope was a 16-residue, proline-rich peptide and part of the repeating region of the CS protein, while the T epitope was a 12-residue amphipathic peptide. The primary or secondary

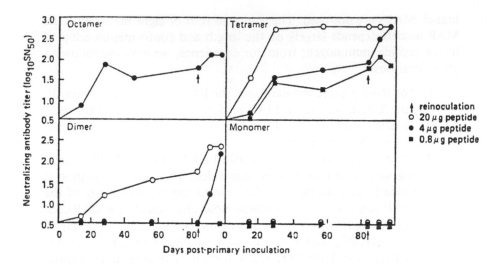

Figure 11 Effect of number of branches and the neutralizing antibody response of guinea pig inoculated IM with mono-, di-, tetra-, and octameric FMDV VP1 141-160 peptides at doses ranging from 20 to 0.8 μg.

antibody responses obtained from A/J mice showed that the tetrameric MAP in the B-T configuration (B epitope as the amino portion connecting to the carboxyl T epitope) was significantly better than the octameric MAP in the same configuration. However, the responses of the tetrameric and octameric MAPs of the opposite orientation (T-B configuration, T epitope as the amino portion connecting to the carboxyl T epitope) were rather similar. As expected, the antibody responses to the MAP construct with the branching in the B-T configuration was 10-fold better than those to the same MAP construct with the T-B configuration because the B epitope occupied the distal and antigenic site (see the previous section, "Antigenic Sites and Monospecific Antibodies"). Thus, these experiments show that the conformation of peptides is a determining factor in the antibody response, and that MAPs containing peptides longer than 24 residues may be more suitable in the four-branch than the eight-branch configuration.

APPLICATIONS TO VACCINES

Requirement of B- and T-Cell Epitopes

A mechanism to generate protective vaccination against infection is the production of neutralizing antibodies. However, the peptide antigen that carries only the neutralizing epitope (the B-cell epitope) may not be sufficiently immunogenic. For this purpose, the B-cell epitope is often conjugated to a protein carrier to enhance its immunogenicity. The carrier thus serves a T-helper-cell function that helps the proliferation of the plasma cells to secrete antibodies of the desired specificity. Since the dominant T-helper-cell epitope can be identified, a major goal toward the development of synthetic peptide vaccines using the MAP approach is the design of suitable models for incorporating the neutralizing B-cell epitope and the dominant T-helper-cell epitope in an optimal arrangement, orientation, and stoichiometry. In the following examples, several MAP models containing both B and T epitopes are used to illustrate the versatility of the oligomeric lysine core matrix for this purpose.

Enhancement of Immunogenicity in a Di-Epitope MAP Against Hepatitis

The major surface antigen (S protein) of HBV (HBsAg) is derived from the S gene, which encodes for a 226-residue protein (49-51). The S protein is processed from two minor but larger envelope proteins, the middle proteins, which contain, in addition to the entire amino acid sequence of the S protein, an NH_2 terminal fragment, the 55-residue pre-S(2), and a 108-119-residue pre-S(1) whose length depends on the strain of HBV. The pre-S(1) region is located upstream from the pre-S(2) region, irrespective of subtypes. The virus-neutralizing antibodies are elicited by the S region of the HBsAg as well as the pre-(S) region of the HBV (51,52).

The majority of anti-HB responses of HBsAg in man, based on serological typing, are against one common group-specific determinant (**a**), which is localized at residues 139-147 of the S protein (52). However, the peptide antigen based on the **a** determinant is a poor immunogen and produces universally low immunological responses in animals (53-55). To overcome this problem, other peptide antigens of the pre-S regions have been investigated, and it has been reported that a peptide of the pre-S(2) protein (residues 14-32) is highly immunogenic (56-58). More importantly, it raises protective antibodies in chimpanzees (57). Thus, these two epitopes of the HBsAg become suitable target peptide antigens for the design of diepitope MAP models. These two peptides were designated as TN-14, a 14-residue peptide representing a tandemly repeating seven-residue peptide of residues 140-146 of the **a** determinant of the S region, and LG-15, a 15-residue peptide of the pre-S(2) protein covering residues 12-26. The antigen LG-15 or TN-14 was synthesized as an acetylated form in an octabranching MAP format (Figure 12). While LG-15 represents a continuous

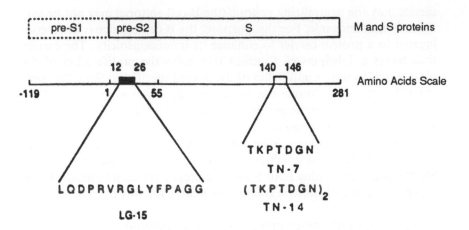

Figure 12 Schematic representation of surface antigens of hepatitis B.

segment of the pre-S(2) sequence, TN-14 represented two tandemly repeating segments of residues 140-146 of the S region (two cysteines normally occurring at positions 139 and 147 were avoided to simplify the
synthesis). The design of tandemly repeating segments of TN-14 would
compensate for the disparity in length between LG-15 (a 15-residue peptide) and the sequence of 140-146 of the S region (a seven-residue peptide).

Two general designs were explored that would incorporate these two
epitopes (Figures 13, 14). In the first design (Figure 13), a cysteinyl dipeptide containing an S-acetamido (Acm) protecting group on the cysteine at
the carboxyl terminus of the MAP was used to form a heterodimer of
either LG-15 or TN-14 MAPs in an end-to-end formation of two octameric

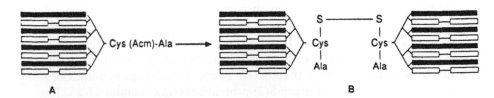

Figure 13 Design of MAP to incorporate two epitopes.

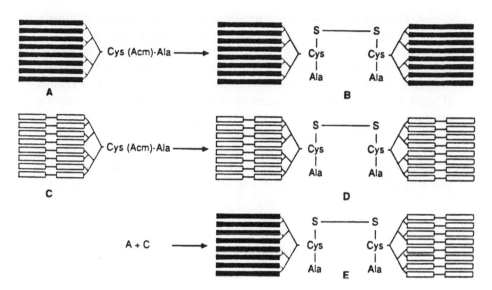

Figure 14 Design of MAP to incorporate two epitopes in alternating form.

MAPs containing the epitopes from S and pre-S(2) regions. This was accomplished by making use of the S-Acm protecting group of the cysteinyl dipeptide and the ability of deblocking and concomitant oxidative actions by I_2 on the S-Acm protecting group (59). When the LG-15 and TN-14 MAPs were mixed in an equal molar ratio, oxidative disulfide formation by I_2 produced a heterodimer containing a diepitope MAP. The oxidation reaction was not quantitative and required purification of the desired heterodimer from the homodimers by gel permeation chromatography.

In the second design, two epitopes were connected in alternating form on the core matrix. However, the design of the cysteinyl dipeptide at the carboxyl terminus was also incorporated. Four copies of two different antigens were attached to the same octabranching MAP to give a diepitope MAP with a design of alternating antigens (Figure 14). The key to the synthesis of this type of MAP was to use an orthogonal protecting group approach in the synthesis of each antigen so that when the synthesis of one antigen was completed, the synthesis of another antigen could be achieved without affecting the integrity of the first antigen. Usually, a combination of two sets of protecting groups—Fmoc/Bu^t and Boc/benzyl—were used.

Antibodies from New Zealand white rabbits immunized with each of the seven MAP models emulsified with complete Freund's adjuvant were tested after 7 weeks for titers reactive with their respective MAPs, the monomeric peptides LG15 or TN14, or with recombinant S and middle proteins. The antibody response could be classified into three groups (Figure 15). The first group, monoepitope LG15 MAP, elicited strong antibody response with titers at about 1:10⁴ dilution to LG15 MAP, the synthetic peptide LG15, and the middle protein consisting of the pre-S(2) and S regions, but not to TN14 MAP or S protein. The second group, monoepitope TN14 MAPs, elicited no response to TN14 MAPs, the monomeric synthetic peptide TN14, or the S protein consisting only of the S

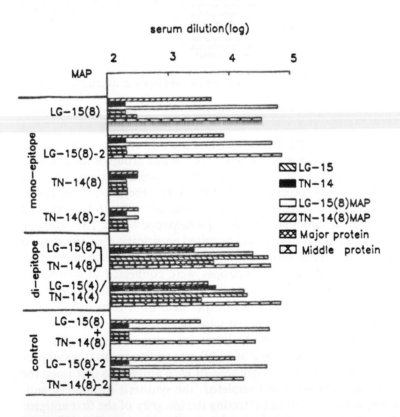

Figure 15 Immune responses of mono- and diepitope MAPs from the S and pre-S(2) antigens.

region, or to the LG15 antigens. The third group, the diepitope MAPs, consisting of covalently linked epitopes, elicited the strongest response with titers at about 1 to 10^5 dilution, to synthetic peptides TN14 and LG15, and both S and middle proteins. Thus, the diepitope MAPs overcame the poor immunogenicity of TN14 and elicited antibody responses to both antigens. The nonresponsiveness of the animals immunized with the TN14 MAPs could not be overcome with a noncovalent mixture consisting of various combinations of monoepitope MAPs of TN14 and LG15. The secondary antibody response after boosting with MAPs did not result in any change in the pattern observed in the primary responses. The mono-epitope MAPs of TN14 produced no significant antibody response, while the diepitope MAPs continued to elicit antibody responses to both deter-minants at about five- to 10-fold higher than those of the primary titers. Similar results were obtained from antibodies obtained after the second and third boosts at 3-week intervals.

The antibodies obtained from the diepitope MAPs were found to be specific, as shown in the immunoblot in SDS polyacrylamide electro-phoresis. These antibodies recognized the HBsAg containing the S region or HBsAg containing both pre-S(2) and S region. Neither preimmune antisera nor the antiLG15 MAP antisera resulted in any reaction. How-ever, anti-TN14 MAP antisera weakly recognized the denatured major and middle proteins. Preincubation of the diepitope MAP antisera with the corresponding synthetic peptide TN14 or LG15 abolished the recogni-tion.

The design of a peptide-based synthetic vaccine requires the inclu-sion of relevant epitopes. Thus, we selected two HB epitopes, the a-deter-minant from the S region and residues 12-26 of the pre-S(2) region. The results show the flexibility and versatility of the MAP approach to in-corporate these epitopes in a chemically defined manner. Furthermore, we also show that the diepitope arrangements result in enhanced immune responses of the a-determinant. The immunogenicity and protective effi-cacy of antibodies elicited by the pre-S(2) region have been taken into consideration in the design of the diepitope MAP models. Indeed, peptide antigens from the pre-S region have been shown to be highly immuno-genic and offer protection to HBV in the chimpanzee models (57). Fur-thermore, the pre-S region is highly conserved, and its peptide antigen efficiently prevents infection against all strains of the four subtypes. More-over, the pre-S region is absent from the present subunit recombinant vaccine, and this provides a strong basis for its inclusion in the synthetic peptide vaccine.

Malaria

Each year, 200 million people are afflicted by malaria, with a fatality rate of 1-2%. Malaria is stage-specific, and the first stage of the malaria parasitic cycle in humans is the sporozoites, which are injected into the host bloodstream by the mosquito. A vaccine against the sporozoite stage appears to be most advantageous to block infection in humans and to prevent transmission of the disease. However, the development of such a vaccine is limited by several technical factors. These factors include the difficulty of obtaining large amounts of the surface antigens of the sporozoites: Malaria is species-specific, and it has been difficult to culture sporozoites specific in infecting humans. A synthetic vaccine based on peptides appears to be most attractive, since the technology is relatively simple and could be transferred to the countries most affected by malaria.

An important requirement for synthetic peptide vaccine is the identification of appropriate B- and T-cell epitopes, so that they may be attached to the MAP system for experimental verification of its efficacy as a vaccine in a well-defined animal model for a specific infectious disease. These requirements can be met in malaria, which is particularly suitable for synthetic vaccine development because no immunophylaxis has yet been developed. Previously, it has been shown that protective immunity against rodent, simian, and human malaria sporozoites can be induced by immunization with irradiated sporozoites (60). The major surface protein of sporozoites is the circumsporozoite (CS) protein, and antibodies directed against the CS portion neutralize the infectivity of the parasites and inhibit their entry into hepatocytes (61). Thus, the CS protein has become a logical choice for the development of vaccines against the sporozoite stage of malaria (62,63). The B-cell epitope of the CS protein of the rodent malaria *Plasmodium berghei* is contained within the repeating domain (64) of the CS protein, a feature common to CS protein of all malaria species (65,66). Mice immunized with a synthetic vaccine consisting of the B epitope attached to tetanus toxoid as a carrier have developed high antibody titers against the native CS protein and resistance to challenge with 10^3 sporozoites (67). However, vaccination attempts in humans, using a similar approach, have failed to induce good antibody titers. This result points to the limitation of using a protein carrier (tetanus toxoid) that leads to epitopic suppression caused by the strong immune response to the carrier protein (68).

Recently, several T-helper-cell epitopes of the CS protein of *P. berghei* have been identified (69), thus providing the opportunity to incorporate B and T epitopes in the MAP models and test their efficacy in a rodent malaria model. We have designed and synthesized 10 models of MAPs containing T- and B-cell epitopes derived from the amino acid sequence of the CS protein of *P. berghei*. The results obtained with the MAP models are compared with those obtained by immunization with the monomeric peptide and with earlier results obtained by immunization with the recombinant protein and irradiated sporozoites of this plasmodial species.

The immunodominant B-cell epitope of the CS protein of *P. berghei* can be represented by a tandemly repeating peptide of 16 residues (Figure 16). A peptide that contains a T-helper-cell epitope recognized by mice of four different H-2 haplotypes is contained between residues 265 and 276 of the CS protein. These T and B epitopes of the CS protein were incorporated into 10 MAP models (Figure 16). The B- and T-helper-cell epitopes are connected in tandem at the core matrix in several arrangements and stoichiometric ratios. These include two models containing four or eight tandemly connecting B and T epitopes [models BT(4) and BT(8)] and two others containing similar epitopes but with the orientation of the B and T epitopes reversed [models TB(4) and TB(8)]. Two models contain different stoichiometry of the B- and T-cell epitopes. B(8)T contains eight copies of the B epitope and only one copy of the T epitope, while model T(8)B contains eight copies of the T epitope and only one copy of the B. As controls, four models of MAPs containing either B- or T-cell epitopes alone in either the tetrameric or octameric arrangement. For comparison, the monomeric model containing only one copy each of the B and T epitopes is also included. Earlier experiments have shown that immunization with the *P. berghei* B-cell epitope alone, either as a monomer (i.e., the 16-residue peptide) or as an octameric MAP, did not elicit antibody responses in several inbred strains of mice bearing different H-2^a haplotypes. This genetic restriction was overcome by the addition of a T helper to the B-cell epitope. For example, A/J mice (H-2^a) did not respond to the octameric MAP containing the B epitope. However, A/J mice that had been primed with a single dose of *P. berghei* sporozoites produced a very strong secondary response when boosted with a synthetic peptide containing in tandem the B epitope and the 265-276 T epitope. Thus, only the diepitope MAP models containing both T- and B-cell epitopes covalently are expected to produce immunological responses in the inbred-strain A/J mice, and the monoepitope MAPs are used as controls.

Groups of five mice of the H-2^a haplotypes (A/J strain) were each immunized with one of the 10 models of MAPs containing the B and T epitopes of the *P. berghei* CS protein. Controls were immunized with the BT monomer, or with a mixture consisting of an equimolar ratio of B(8)

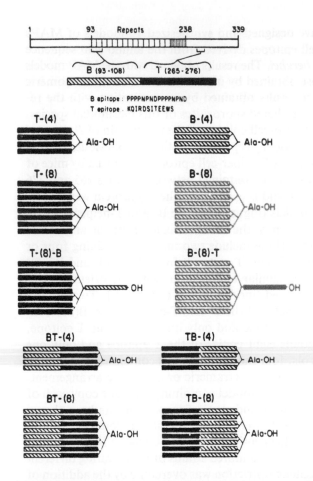

Figure 16 Structure of the CS protein, the monomeric form of a peptide containing both the tandem connecting B- and T-cell epitopes of *P. berghei*, and schematic representation of 10 MAP models. For convenience, each model is named by the shortened form of (epitopes)-(number of branching); e.g., T-(4) is depicted in the first MAP model.

and T(8). The sera obtained from each group of animals were pooled and assayed for their reactivity with the recombinant CS protein (IRMA) and with glutaraldehyde-fixed sporozoites by indirect immunofluorescence assay (IFA).

Based on the antibody responses 3 weeks following the first antigen dose, the MAPs could be classified into two groups according to their immunogenicity (Figure 17). The MAPs which contained equimolar amounts of T and B epitopes, linked in tandem, were highly immunogenic and elicited high antibody titers. The best immunogen, BT(4), produced serum antibody levels detectable at dilutions greater than 10^5, and the others induced serum titers between 6.4×10^4 and 2.5×10^4. The poorly immunogenic MAPs included the two in which there were different ratios of B and T epitopes [B(8)T and T(8)B]. B(4) and B(8) were nonimmunogenic as expected because they did not contain a T-helper epitope to overcome the genetic restriction of the immune response in A/J mice. There was a very poor antibody response to T(4) and T(8) or to TB monomers. Thus, a covalent high-molecular-weight structure containing multiple copies of both B and T epitopes such as BT(4) or TB(4) was required for

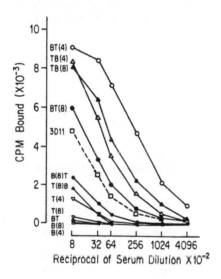

Figure 17 Secondary antibody responses of groups of mice immunized with different MAP models. Groups of five mice of the H-2^a halotype (B10.A strain) were injected IP with 50 μg of each MAP or a mixture of MAPs [T-(8) + B-(8)], emulsified in CFA on day 0, and boosted with 50 μg of the same antigen in IFA on day 21. Sera were collected 21 days later. Sera were pooled and antibody titers determined by an immunodiometric assay using recombinant protein as a solid-phase antigen. The titers were expressed as the reciprocal of the highest positive serum dilution. For comparison, the titers of sporozoite (3D11) were also shown (broken lines).

immunogenicity since the mixture of equimolar amounts of B(8) and T(8) failed to elicit any antibody responses.

In general, the antibody responses observed 21 and 34 days after a second dose of the MAPs were significantly higher, but the ranking order of immunogenicity was similar to that observed in the primary responses. The most immunogenetic MAP, BT(4), produced antibodies that reacted at serum dilutions of 5×10^5, while the other three diepitope MAPs, containing equimolar amounts of T and B, produced titers between 100,000 and 400,000. Animals immunized with the monoepitope MAPs, such as B(4) and B(8) MAPs, remained nonresponders. The immunofluorescence (IFA) titers of the sera 34 days after the booster injection are shown in Table 1. The BT(4)-injected mice had IFA titers of 128×10^3, which are much higher than the $5\text{-}15 \times 10^3$ IFA titers usually found in the serum of mice hyperimmunized with irradiated sporozoites. Immunization of A/J mice with similar doses of recombinant *P. berghei* CS protein, encompassing amino acids 81-277, resulted in much lower IFA titers (2×10^3).

Table 1 Protective Efficacy of Different MAP Models in Mice Challenged with 2000 *P. berghei* Sporozoites

Immunogen[a]	Antisporozoite[b] IFA titer $\times 10^{-3}$	Number[c] protected/challenged	Protection (%)
BT-MAP(4)	128	4/5	80
TB-MAP(4)	32	3/5	60
TB-MAP(8)	32	3/5	60
BT-MAP(8)	8	2/4	50
T-MAP(4)	<0.2	0/4	0
B-MAP(4)	<0.2	0/5	0
B-MAP(8)	<0.2	0/5	0
BT monomer	<0.2	0/5	0
No immunogen	—	0/5	0

[a]Structures of different immunogens. See Figure 16.
[b]Titer determined by IFA (indirect immunofluorescence assay) fixed sporozoites 1 week before challenge and represented the highest reactive dilution.
[c]Mice were challenged by intravenous inoculations of 2000 sporozoites 35 days after the second immunizing dose. Peripheral blood smears were examined for parasitized erythrocytes 1 and 2 weeks after challenge.

The apparent greater immunogenicity of BT(4) than that of other di-epitope models appears to be consistent with the general conclusion derived from the previous discussion (see "Characteristics of Immune Responses" above). BT(4) contains the favorable B epitope at the distal end of the MAP construct and the less crowded tetrameric format when the immunogen is long (BT = 28 residues). In the present case, the less bulky model BT(4) produced about 50-fold higher antibody titers than BT(8). On the other hand, there is little difference in response between the reversely oriented models TB(8) and BT(8). The B-cell epitope of the CS protein is exceptionally rich in proline (50%), while the T-cell epitope has a strong propensity for amphipathic helix formation. Although the present results indicate that there is no advantage to increasing the number of MAP branches from four to eight, the effects on the immune response of the number and orientation of the B- and T-cell epitopes in the MAP models may be sequence-dependent and may require optimization in a given experimental system.

The efficacy of the MAPs as a vaccine was determined by an intravenous challenge with 2000 *P. berghei* sporozoites 35 days after the secondary immunization with MAPs. In the group of mice immunized with BT(4), 80% of the mice were protected, while in the group of mice immunized with the other three diepitope MAPs, there was 50 to 60% protection (Table 1). No protection was observed with the mice immunized with the monoepitope MAPs. The antisporozoite antibody levels, as determined by IFA before the challenge, correlated well with the degree of protection.

A synthetic *P. falciparum* malaria vaccine consisting of (NANP)₃, the B-cell epitope of the CS protein, coupled to the tetanus toxoid carrier, has undergone human trials (70). The frequency and magnitude of the antibody response to the peptide increased with the dose of antigen. However, due to the toxicity of tetanus toxoid, the vaccine dose could not be increased. One of the disappointing findings of this trial was that the antibody levels were much lower than those in mice given the same vaccine. In part this may be due to the relatively high dose of the conjugate given to mice, or because the human volunteers had been vaccinated with tetanus toxoid, and their response to the B-cell epitope was therefore inhibited by antibodies to the tetanus toxoid. The diepitope MAPs should overcome both the problems of epitopic suppression and carrier toxicity. Furthermore, the MAPs are chemically defined, contain a high density of epitopes, and, as shown here, can produce high levels of parasite-specific protective antibodies.

CONCLUDING REMARKS

In this paper, I have described a new approach, MAP, for the preparation of peptide-based immunogens and synthetic vaccines. The central thesis of this approach is the use of a low-molecular-weight core matrix as a replacement of the protein carrier, and the key element is the design of this low-molecular-weight (<900 dalton), branching lysine core matrix that is used as a framework connecting the same or different peptide immunogens in a desired arrangement and orientation. In this way, the preparation of the peptide immunogens becomes quantitative and chemically unambiguous.

In laboratory use, MAPs containing peptides of 10 to 20 amino acids are found to be highly immunogenic and elicit monospecific antibodies in a controlled response in animals. The required peptide immunogens in the MAP approach are in general longer than those in the conventional approach because part of the peptide also serves the T-helper activity. The major antigenic site of these antigens is found at the flexible end of the peptide, distal to the end attached to the core matrix.

For the preparation of experimental synthetic vaccine, a distinct advantage of the design of MAP is the flexibility of engineering copies of both B and T epitopes in a defined manner. The involvement of the cell-mediated immune response becomes an important factor for enhancement and specific memory of immunogenicity, cell replication, and differentiation of antibody after stimulation. The importance of incorporating a predetermined, dominant T-helper-cell epitope becomes evident when the antibody responses of the mono- and diepitopes of MAP models in the hepatitis and malaria vaccines are compared. Monoepitope MAPs containing only the B-cell epitopes are poor immunogens. On the contrary, diepitope MAPs containing both B- and T-cell epitopes have enhanced immune responses, produce high neutralizing antibody titers, and provide significant protective immunity against infectivity in the mouse malaria model.

One of the functions of protein carriers such as serum albumin, keyhole limpet hemocyanin, or tetanus toxoid is often to enhance the immunogenicity of the synthetic peptides by providing a T-helper-cell epitope. However, such carriers are not suitable for use in human vaccines. The inclusion of a protein carrier, besides the disadvantage of chemical ambiguity, can lead to the complications of hypersensitivity to the carrier and epitopic suppression. Thus, it appears that the MAP approach containing the T-cell-helper epitope eliminates the need of a protein carrier.

One of the strengths of the synthetic peptide vaccine lies in its conceptual simplicity that allows rational design to give the desired selective immune responses. However, this minimalistic strategy is a challenge that requires the basic understanding of the nature of the infectious organism and the immunity required for its protection. The MAP approach is likely to facilitate such a challenge and holds the future promise of functioning as a synthetic peptide vaccine.

ACKNOWLEDGMENTS

This work was supported in part by US PHS AI 28701 and from AID OGAS 122. I sincerely thank Drs. D. N. Posnett, P. Clavijo, Y. A. Lu, V. Nussenzweig, R. Nussenzweig, and F. Zavala for their contributions to this work.

REFERENCES

1. Ada GL. Modern vaccines. The immunological principles of vaccination. Lancet 1990; 335:523-526.
2. Brown F. Modern vaccines. From Jenner to genes—the new vaccines. Lancet 1990; 335:587-590.
3. Milich DR. Synthetic T and B cell recognition sites: implications for vaccine development. Adv Immunol 1989; 45:195-282.
4. Sela M. Antigencity: some molecular aspects. Science 1969; 166:1465-1474.
5. Arnon R, Maron E, Sela M, Anfinsen CB. Antibodies reactive with native lysozyme elicited by a completely synthetic antigen. Proc Natl Acad Sci USA 1971; 68:1450-1455.
6. Sutcliffe JG, Shinnick TM, Green N, Lerner R. Antibodies that react with predetermined sites on proteins. Science 1983; 219:660-666.
7. Walter G, Scheidtman K, Carbone A, Laudano AP, Doolittle RF. Antibodies specific for the carboxy- and amino-terminal regions of simian virus 40 large tumor antigen. Proc Natl Acad Sci USA 1980; 77:5197-5201.
8. DiMarchi R, Brooke G, Gale C, Cracknell V, Doel T, Mowat N. Protection of cattle against foot-and-mouth disease by a synthetic peptide. Science 1986; 232:639-641.
9. Jacob CO, Arnon R, Sela M. Effect of carrier on the immunogenic capacity of synthetic cholera vaccine. Mol Immunol 1985; 22:1333-1339.
10. Nussenzweig V, Nussenzweig RS. Adv Immunol 1989; 45:283.
11. Tam JP. Synthetic peptide vaccine design: Synthesis and properties of a high-density multiple antigen peptide system. Proc Natl Acad Science USA 1988; 85:5409-5413.

12. Tam JP. A high-density multiple antigen peptide system for the preparation of antipeptide antibodies. In: Michael Conn P, ed. Hormone Action. Part I. Methods in Enzymology: Neuroendocrine Peptide Methodology. San Diego, CA: Academic Press, 1988:619-627.

13. Francis MJ, Hastings GZ, Brown F, McDermed J, Lu YA, Tam JP. Immunological evaluation of the multiple antigen peptide (MAP) system using the major immunogenic site of foot-and-mouth disease virus. Immunol 1991. In press.

14. Chang KJ, Pugh W, Blanchard SG, McDermed J, Tam JP. Antibody specific to α-subunit of guanine nucleotide binding regulatory protein, G_o: Development and immunocytochemical localization of α_o in brain. Proc Natl Acad Sci USA 1988; 86:4929-4933.

15. Zavala F, Romero PJ, Ley V, Nussenzweig R, Nussenzweig V, Tam JP, Barr PJ. Synthetic peptide vaccine against murine malaria. In: Vaccines '88. Cold Spring Harbor, NY: Cold Spring Harbor Laboratories 1988; 6:66-70.

16. Posnett D, McGrath H, Tam J. A novel method for producing anti-peptide antibodies using a peptide derived from the T cell antigen receptor β-chain constant region. J Biol Chem 1988; 263:1719-1725.

17. Tam JP, Zavala F. Multiple antigen peptide: A novel approach to increase sensitivity for the detection of synthetic peptide antigens in solid phase immunoassays. J Immunol Meth 1989; 124:53-61.

18. Tam JP. Multiple antigen peptide system. A novel design for synthetic peptide vaccine and immunoassay. In: Tam JP, Kaiser ET, eds. Synthetic Peptides: Approaches to Biological Problems. New York: Alan R Liss, 1989: 3-18.

19. Tam JP. Multiple antigen peptide system: A novel design for peptide-based vaccines. In: Chanock R, Brown F, Lerner R, Ginsberg H, eds. Vaccines '89. Cold Spring Harbor, NY: Cold Spring Harbor Laboratories, 1989:21-25.

20. Tam JP, Clavijo P, Lu YA, Nussenzweig RS, Nussenzweig V, Zavala F. Incorporation of T and B epitopes of the circumsporozoite protein in a chemically defined synthetic vaccine against malaria. J Exp Med 1990; 171:299-306.

21. Tam JP, Lu YA. Vaccine engineering: Enhancement of immunogenicity of synthetic peptide vaccines related to hepatitis in chemically defined models consisting of T and B cell epitopes. Proc Natl Acad Sci USA 1989; 86:9084-9008.

22. Schaaper WMM, Lu YA, Tam JP, Meloen RH. Fine specificity of antisera raised against a multiple antigenic peptide from foot-and-mouth disease virus. In: Rivier JE, Marshall GR, eds. Peptides: Chemistry, Structure and Biology. Lethen, Netherlands: ESCOM Science Publishers, 1990:765-766.

23. Tam JP, Lu YA. Synthetic peptide vaccine engineering: Design and synthesis of unambiguous peptide-based vaccines containing multiple peptide antigens for malaria and hepatitis. In: Epton R, ed. Innovation and Perspectives

in Solid Phase Synthesis—Peptides, Polypeptides and Oligonucleotides: Macro-organic Reagents and Catalysts. Bermingham, England: SPCC (UK), 1990:351-370.

24. Lu YA, Clavijo P, Galantino M, Shen ZY, Liu W, Tam JP. Chemically unambiguous peptide immunogen: Preparation, orientation, and antigenicity of purified peptide conjugated to the multiple antigen peptide system. Mol Immunol 1991; 28:623-630.

25. Clavijo P, Lu YA, Nussenzweig R, Cochrane A, Zavala F, Nardin E, Tam JP. Immunogenicity of MAPS containing B and T cell epitopes of a malarial antigen, the circumsporozoite protein. In: Proceedings of the 21st European Peptide Symposium. Platja D'Aro, Spain. 1990:839-842.

26. Zavala F, Tam JP, Masuda A. Synthetic peptides as antigens for the detection of humoral immunity to *Plasmodium falciparum* Sporozoites. J Immunol Methods 1986; 93:55-61.

27. Merrifield RB. Solid phase synthesis. Science 1986; 232:341-347.

28. Merrifield RB. Solid phase synthesis. I. The synthesis of a terapeptide. J Am Chem Soc 1963; 85:2149-2154.

29. Tam JP, Heath WF, Merrifield RB. S_N2 Deprotection of synthetic peptides with a low concentration of HF in dimethyl sulfide: Evidence and application in peptide synthesis. J Am Chem Soc 1983; 105:6442.

30. Linder W, Robey FA. Automated synthesis and use of N-chloroacetyl-modified peptides for the preparation of synthetic peptide polymers and peptide protein immunogens. Int J Pept Prot Res 1987; 30:794-800.

31. Robey FA, Fields RL. Automated synthesis of N-bromoacetyl-modified peptide for the preparation of synthetic peptide polymers, peptide-protein conjugates, and cyclic peptides. Anal Biochem 1989; 177:373-377.

32. Avrameas S, Ternyck T. The cross-linking of proteins with glutaraldehyde and its use for the preparation of immunosorbents. Immunochem 1969; 6:53-66.

33. Bernatowicz MS, Matsueda GR. Preparation of peptide-protein immunogens using N-succinimidy bromo acetate as a heterobifunctional crosslinking reagent. Anal Biochem 1986; 155:95-102.

34. Lee A, Powell JE, Tregar GW, Niall H, Stevens V. A method for preparing β HCG COOH peptide-carrier conjugates of predictable composition. Mol Immunol 1980; 17:749-756.

35. Kitagawa T, Aikawa T. Enzyme coupled immunoassay of insulin using a novel coupling reagent. J Biochem 1976; 79:233-236.

36. Yoshitake S, Yamada Y, Ishikawa E, Masseyeff R. Conjugation of glucose oxidase from *Aspergillus niger* and rabbit antibodies using N-hydroxysuccinimide ester of N-(4-carboxycyclohexylmethyl)-maleimide. Eur J Biochem 1979; 101:395-399.

37. Martin FJ, Papahadjopoulos D. Irreversible coupling of immunoglobulin fragments of preformed vesicles. J Biol Chem 1982; 257:286-288.

38. Carlsson J, Drevin H, Axen R. Protein thiolation and reversible protein-protein conjugation. N-succinimidyl 3-(2-pyridyldithio)propionate, a new heterobifunctional reagent. Biochemistry 1978; 173:723-737; 158, 1570-1572.

39. Dyrberg T, Oldstone MB. Peptides as antigens: Importance of orientation. J Exp Med 1986; 164:1344-1349.

40. Tam JP. Synthesis of biologically active transforming growth factor alpha. Int J Pept Prot Res 1987; 29:421-431.

41. Geysen HM, Meloen RH, Berteling SJ. Use of peptide synthesis to probe viral antigens for epitopes to a resolution of a single amino acid. Proc Natl Acad Sci 1984; 81:3998-4002.

42. Rosenthal AS. Immunological Rev 1978; 40:135-152.

43. Good MF, Pombo D, Quakyi I, Riley E, Houghten RA, Menon A, et al. Human T-cell recognition of the circumsporozoite protein of plasmodium faciparum: Immunodominant T-cell domains MAP to the polymorphic regions of the molecule. Proc Natl Acad Sci USA 1988; 85:1199-1203.

44. Allen PM, Strydom DJ, Unanue ER. Processing of lysozyme by macrophages: identification of the determinant by two T-cell hybridomas. Proc Natl Acad Sci USA 1984; 81:2489-2493.

45. Buus S, Sette A, Colon SM, Miles C, Grey HM. The relation between major histocompatibility complex (MHC) restriction and the capacity of Ia to bind immunogenic peptide. Science 1987; 235:1353-1358.

46. Celis E, Chang TW. Antibodies to hepatitis B surface antigen potentiate the response of human T lymphocyte clones to the same antigen. Science 1984; 224:297-299.

47. Delisi C, Berzofsky JA. T-cell antigenic sites tend to be amphipathic structures. Proc Natl Acad Sci USA 1985; 82:7048-7052.

48. Good MF, Maloy WL, Lunde MN, Margalit H, Cornette JL, Smith GL, et al. Construction of synthetic immunogen: Use of new T-helper epitope on malarial cirumsporozoite protein science 1987; 235:1059-1062.

49. Tiollais P, Charnay P, Vyas GN. Biology of hepatitis B virus. Science 1981; 213:406-411.

50. Tiollais P, Pourcel C, Dejean A. The hepatitis B virus. Nature 1985; 317: 489-495.

51. Valenzuela P, Quiroga M, Zaldivar J, Gray P, Rutter WJ. In: Fields B, Jaenisch R, Fox CF, eds. Animal Virus Genetics. New York: Academic Press, 1980: 57-70.

52. Stevens CE, Alter HJ, Taylor PE, Zhng EA, Harley EJ, Szmuness W. Hepatitis B vaccine in patients receiving hemodialysis. N Engl J Med 1984; 311:496.

53. Purcell RH, Gerin JL. Prospects for second and third generation hepatitis B vaccine. Hepatology 1985; 5:159-163.

54. Bhatnagar PK, Papas E, Blum HE, Milich DR, Nitecki D, Karels MJ, Vyas GN. Immune response to synthetic peptide analogues of hepatitis B surface antigen specific for the A determinant. Proc Natl Acad Sci USA 1982; 79: 4400-4404.

55. Prince AM, Ikram H, Hopp T. Hepatitis B virus vaccine: Identification of HBsAg/a and HBsAg/d but not HBsAg/y subtype antigenic determinants on a synthetic immunogenic peptide. Proc Natl Acad Sci USA 1982; 79:579-582.

56. Neurath AR, Kent SBH, Strick N. Science 1984; 224:392-395. Neurath RA, Kent SBH. Adv Virus Res 1988; 34:65-135.

57. Itoh Y, Takai E, Ohnuma H, Kitajima K, Tsuda F, Machida A, Mishiro S, Nakamura T, Miyakawa Y, Mayumi M. A synthetic peptide vaccine involving the product of the pre-S(2) region of hepatitis B virus DNA: protective efficacy in chimapanzees. Proc Natl Acad Sci USA 1986; 83:9174-9178.

58. Milich DR, Thornton GB, Neurath AR, Kent SBH, Michel ML, Tiollais P, Chisari F. Enhanced immunogenicity of the pre-S region of hepatitis B surface antigen. Science 1985; 228:1195-1199.

59. Veber S, Milkowski JD, Varga SL, Denkewalter RG, Hirschmann R. J Am Chem Soc 1972; 94:5456-5461.

60. Yoshida N, Nussenzweig RS, Potocnjak P, Nussenzweig V, Aikawa M. Hybridoma produces protective antibodies directed against the sporozoite stage of malaria parasites. Science 1980; 207:71-73.

61. Egan JE, Weber JL, Ballou WR, Hollingdale MR, Majarian WR, et al. Efficacy of murine malaria sporozoite vaccine: Implications for human vaccine development. Science 1987; 236:453.

62. Zavala F, Tam JP, Hollingdale MR, Cochrane AH, Quakyi I, Nussenzweig RS, Nussenzweig V. Rationale for development of a synthetic vaccine against *Plasmodium falciparum* malaria. Science 1985; 228:1436-1440.

63. Ballou WR, Hoffman SL, Sherwood JA, Hollingdale MR, Neva FA, Hockmeyer WT, Gordon DM, Schneider I, Wirtz RA, Young JF, Wasserman GF, Reeve P, Diggs CL, Chulay JD. Safety and efficacy of a recombinant DNA *Plasmodium falciparum* sporozoite vaccine. Lancet 1987; 1:1277.

64. Eichinger DJ, Arnot DE, Tam JP, Nussenzweig V, Enea V. Circumsporozoite protein of *Plasmodium berghei*: gene cloning and identification of the immunodominant epitope. Mol Cell Biol 1986; 6:3965.

65. Weber JL, Egan JE, Lyon JA, Wirtz RA, Charoenvit Y, Maloy WL, Hockmeyer WT. Exp Parasitol 1987; 63:295.

66. Dame JB, Williams JL, McCutchan TF, Weber JL, Wirtx RA, Hockmeyer WT, Maloy WL, Haynes JD, Schneider I, Roberts D, Sanders GS, Reddy EP, Diggs CL, Miller LH. Structure of the gene encoding the immunodominant surface antigen on the sporozoite of the human malaria parasite *Plasmodium falciparum*. Science 1984; 225:593-599.

67. Zavala F, Tam JP, Barr PJ, Romero PJ, Ley V, Nussenzweig RS, Nussenzweig V. Synthetic peptide vaccine confers protection against murine malaria. J Exp Med 1987; 166:1591.

68. Herzenberg LA, Tokuhisa T. Epitope-specific regulation. J Exp Med 1983; 155:1730.

69. Romero PJ, Tam JP, Schlesinger D, Clavijo P, Barr PJ, Nussenzweig RS, Nussenzweig V, Zavala F. Multiple T helper cell epitopes of the circumsporozoite protein of *Plasmodium berghei*. Eur J Immunol 1988; 18:1951.

4

The Use of Muramyl Peptides as Vaccine Adjuvants

Gary Ott, Gary Van Nest, and Rae Lyn Burke
Chiron Corporation
Emeryville, California

INTRODUCTION

One of the challenges associated with vaccine development today is the development of safe and effective adjuvants for human administration. The need for effective adjuvants becomes more pronounced as the vaccine field attempts to move from traditional live virus vaccines to the theoretically safer but less immunogenic subunit vaccines that now can be practically and economically produced using recombinant DNA technology. Currently, the only adjuvants approved for human use are the aluminum salts (alum). Alum has been effective for some vaccines, but it has limited immunostimulatory capacity, especially for the stimulation of cellular immune responses. The prototype potent adjuvant is complete Freunds' adjuvant (CFA) (1), consisting of a water-in-oil emulsion containing approximately 50% mineral oil, the emulsifying agent Arlacel A, and killed mycobacterium. While an effective adjuvant, CFA is unacceptable for human use (and undesirable for general animal administration) due to its severe side effects, including pain, abscess formation, local necrosis, and fever. Omission of the mycobacteria generates incomplete Freund's adjuvant (IFA), which reduces both the immune response and the side effects. Side effects associated with IFA, predominantly the formation of granulomas at the site of vaccination, are still considered too severe for general human use. Thus, the goal of adjuvant research in the last 40 years has been to find effective, nontoxic substitutes for both the vehicle (mineral oil and Arlacel A) and the immunostimulatory components (mycobacteria) of CFA while maintaining adjuvant activity.

Many scientists contributed to a dissection of the adjuvant active moieties from the mycobacterial cell wall. The most studied activity, that of muramyl peptides, was characterized by isolating first a wax-soluble derivative (2-4) then a water-soluble peptidoglycan component (5-7). Ellouz and co-workers (8) identified the minimal structure capable of evoking much of the adjuvant activity of the mycobacterial extract as a muramyl dipeptide, N-acetylmuramyl-L-alanyl-D-isoglutamine, or MDP. This compound was subsequently chemically synthesized by Merser et al. (9) and Kotani et al. (10). Since that time, hundreds of different derivatives of muramyl dipeptide have been synthesized in efforts to increase adjuvant potency and decrease toxicity. Simultaneously, a large number of different vehicles have been developed and tested for delivery of antigen and muramyl peptides. These vehicles have included liposomes, water-in-oil (w/o) emulsions, and oil-in-water (o/w) emulsions. In this review we address the use of muramyl peptides as vaccine adjuvants, with a special emphasis on the role of the delivery vehicle for the optimization of the immune responses.

ACTIVITIES ASSOCIATED WITH MURAMYL PEPTIDES

Muramyl peptides have been demonstrated to effect a host of activities on a variety of cell types involved in generating immune responses. The primary target cell of muramyl peptide-mediated adjuvant responses appears to be the macrophage (11). Muramyl peptides are able to activate many macrophage functions, including colloidal carbon clearance (12-15), priming for superoxide production (16,17), spreading and adherence (18), tumoricidal activity (19-21), and release of monokines. The stimulation of macrophage IL-1 production, both secreted (22-24) and membrane-bound forms (25), probably plays a central role in the adjuvant activity of muramyl peptides. Other monokines secreted by macrophages in response to muramyl peptides include TNF [when used in combination with lipopolysaccharide (LPS)] (26,27), CSF (24,28-30), and IL-6 (31). Muramyl peptides have also been demonstrated to induce monocyte proliferation in vivo in guinea pigs and rabbits (32,33) and to increase the number of bone marrow granulocyte-macrophage precursor cells in mice (34).

In addition to macrophages, muramyl peptides also directly stimulate B cells and can substitute for T-cell help, but generally this activity is demonstrable when administered in conjunction with monokines or mitogens. Muramyl peptide was shown to stimulate DNA synthesis in anti-IgM-activated B cells (35), IL-2-stimulated B cells (36), and polyclonally activated B cells (36). Muramyl peptides can stimulate the primary antibody response of macrophage-depleted spleen cells or purified B cells supplemented with monokines (37,38). Similarly, in vitro antibody production from lymph node cells is induced by supernatants from MDP-stimulated macrophages, whereas supernatants from unstimulated macrophages are ineffective (39). The mitogenic activity of a number of MDP derivatives seems to correlate with adjuvant potency. However, it should be noted that MDP is a far less effective B-cell mitogen than other bacterial components, such as LPS, murein, lipopeptides, and lipid A (39).

Muramyl peptides alone do not appear to directly stimulate T cells, but they increase T-cell responses to IL-2, increase IL-2 production in standard mixed lymphocyte culture (MLC), and increase the alloantigen-induced proliferation of T cells in MLC with suboptimal numbers of stimulator cells (39,40). Muramyl peptides can induce T-suppressor cells in mice (41), and T-cell cytolytic activity can be increased by the presence of muramyl peptides in the stimulation phase (39). The induction of delayed-type hypersensitivity to protein antigens is one of the hallmarks of the adjuvant activity of MDPs (8,39,42). In addition, muramyl peptides can induce natural killer-cell activity in mice (43,44) and activate phagocytic and chemotactic activities of polymorphonuclear leukocytes (45). Prophylactic administration of MDP stimulates broad, nonspecific immunity to a variety of bacterial, fungal, and viral infections such as influenza, parainfluenza, and herpesviruses in mice and guinea pigs (15,46-49).

An exact definition of the in vitro or in vivo activities of muramyl peptides responsible for the in vivo adjuvant efficacy is difficult due to the multiple activities associated with these molecules, many of which may contribute to adjuvant effects. Certainly macrophage activation appears to play a central role in muramyl peptide activity. Many other effects are probably secondary responses to macrophage factors induced by the muramyl peptides.

Side Effects

While muramyl peptides appear to be attractive candidates for human vaccine adjuvants, a number of toxic side effects that have been associated with their use in animals must be considered. These side effects include: pyrogenicity, induction of granulomas, adjuvant-induced arthritis, uveitis, necrotic inflammation, and toxic shock. Pyrogenic effects are perhaps the side effects most often associated with muramyl peptides (50-52). Whereas the natural muramyl dipeptide (N-acetylmuramyl-L-alanyl-D-isoglutamine) is pyrogenic, a number of derivatives of muramyl dipeptide have been synthesized that retain adjuvant activity but show reduced pyrogenicity. These derivatives include the butyl ester derivative Murabutide (53), threonyl-MDP (thr-MDP) (54), B30-MDP (55), and MTP-PE (56). Granuloma formation has been associated with the use of muramyl peptides, but this side effect is usually seen only in association with Freund's-like w/o emulsions (57,58) or when conjugated to certain fatty acids (59). Muramyl dipeptides injected in saline induced no granulomas (60). Thus, careful selection of an adjuvant carrier/vehicle for the use of muramyl peptides can probably control the formulation of granulomas.

Adjuvant-induced arthritis, in contrast, has been associated with the use of muramyl peptides with and without oil vehicles (60-63). The ability of different muramyl peptide derivatives to induce arthritis varies widely (63,64). As with the pyrogenicity effects, arthritic effects of eventual vaccine adjuvants can probably be controlled by the correct choice of the muramyl peptide derivative. Induction of uveitis in the rabbit has been demonstrated (65,66) but, as with many of the other side effects, the ability of different muramyl peptides to induce this effect varies. Derivatives demonstrated to have very low uveitis-inducing ability include Murabutide, thr-MDP, and n-butyl-[Val]-MDP (66). Some side effects, including necrotic inflammation and toxic shock, are induced by the combined effects of muramyl peptides and endotoxin. Combinations of muramyl dipeptide, trehalose dimycolate, and endotoxin lead to endotoxic shock, which sometimes results in death in guinea pigs (67), and muramyl peptides amplify the lethal toxicity of LPS in mice (68). In addition, it has been demonstrated that muramyl peptides can cause necrotic reactions in the footpads of guinea pigs previously primed with tubercle bacilli (69). The ability of different muramyl peptides to demonstrate this effect again varied widely. Derivatives that were capable of inducing necrosis in primed guinea pigs were generally powerful adjuvants, but good adjuvant derivatives did not necessarily have necrosis-inducing activity (70).

The association with muramyl peptides of the various side effects discussed above indicates that caution must be used in their application to human vaccines. While some of the side effects noted in the experimental animals are severe, many experiments imply that side effects can be eliminated or significantly reduced by carefully optimizing several parameters for low toxicity. Parameters that must be balanced between efficacy and safety include the choice of the muramyl peptide to be used, the choice of adjuvant vehicle for delivery of adjuvant and antigen, adjuvant dose, and route of delivery. Muramyl peptides that appear most promising from a safety-versus-efficacy consideration include Murabutide, threonyl-MDP, [B30]-MDP, and MTP-PE. Evidence to date would indicate that the use of Freund's-like vehicles with muramyl peptides should be avoided.

VEHICLES FOR MURAMYL PEPTIDE DELIVERY

Multiple carriers have been employed with muramyl dipeptides and their derivatives. These include saline, w/o emulsions (with nearly 50% oil in a w/o emulsion) or o/w emulsions (containing 10% or less oil in o/w emulsions), liposomes, alum, and direct covalent linkage to proteins or peptide-hapten conjugates. Various combinations of these vehicles have also been employed, such as presentation of covalent conjugates bound to alum, linked to liposomes, or in emulsions. Presentation of antigen and muramyl peptide in saline is generally poorly immunogenic and generates antibody and protective immune responses lower than or similar to those obtained with protein absorbed to alum. In general, presentation in saline is insufficiently immunogenic to warrant the risk of side effects. Humoral responses are elevated compared to vaccine without adjuvant, but are similar to those obtained with alum (71) while cellular responses have been reported to be poor (72,73). Many of the early studies employed IFA, a high-oil w/o emulsion as a carrier, thereby demonstrating that MDP could substitute for the mycobacterial cell-wall component of CFA. However, as noted earlier, the side effects of IFA are unacceptable; thus, current research focuses on the use of vehicles with intermediate adjuvant properties and reduced toxicities. These include o/w emulsions, liposomes, and MDP-antigen conjugates.

Oil-in-Water Emulsions

An extensive history of both parenteral and oral administration of o/w emulsions has been documented (74). This type of adjuvant carrier has been derived largely from two basic systems: the parenteral nutrition emulsions, which utilize phospholipids to emulsify safflower or soybean oil (75,76) to form synthetic lipoproteins, and the Ribi system, which utilizes polyoxyethylene sorbitan esters to emulsify squalene (77) and provide the requisite surface for display of trehalose dimycolate (78), lipid A (79), or a variety of other hydrophobic surface agents (80), most notably the pluronic block polymers (81-83).

Muramyl peptides have been used in conjunction with o/w emulsions by several groups. The hydrophilic threonyl MDP derivative has been used extensively with a low-oil emulsion containing 10% squalene, 0.24% Tween-80, and 5% pluronic L121 designated SAF-1 (84). Antibody titers against ovalbumin in guinea pigs were increased 2.4-fold by antigen presentation in SAF-1 vehicle compared to saline and the inclusion of 250 μg threonyl MDP augmented titers an additional 3.6-fold. Delayed-type hypersensitivity was also substantially increased upon addition of the muramyl peptide. In mice and guinea pigs, the same formulation elicited more than a 10-fold increase in antibody titer to influenza B hemagglutinin compared to the saline-formulated vaccine when measured by ELISA, hemagglutination inhibition, or neutralization (85). The antigen dose could be decreased 10-fold in the vaccine containing adjuvant without a significant change in titer. In "elderly" mice (who respond very weakly to hemagglutinin in saline), the use of the SAF-1 formulation gave about a 50-fold increase in ELISA titer. This combination of muramyl dipeptide derivative and o/w emulsion has been reported to have low toxicity and minimal side effects.

The use of hydrophobic MDP derivatives that associate directly with the surface of oil droplets has been reported by two groups. B30-MDP has been used as an adjuvant for ovalbumin with a series of vehicles including a Ribi-like squalene/water emulsion and an intralipidlike phospholipid-emulsified soy oil formulation (86). Antibody titers increased 1.5-2-fold with the addition of B30-MDP in either the squalene/water or intralipidlike formulations compared to saline. Incorporation of a soluble or hydrophilic derivative of MDP did not enhance the immunogenicity of an intralipidlike emulsion. These B30-MDP formulations elicited titers in guinea pigs equal to or greater than those achieved with B30-MDP in a Freund's-like high-oil emulsion and about twofold higher than that obtained with unilamellar liposomes. The delayed-type hypersensitivity response was greatest for the o/w vehicle. Swelling at the injection site was substantially reduced with o/w versus w/o formulations. The relative swelling of regional lymph nodes was antigen dose-dependent. At high antigen doses, the o/w formulations provoked more pronounced enlargement of the nodes.

The hydrophobic muramyl peptide derivative MTP-PE has been combined with a recombinant herpes simplex virus (HSV) glycoprotein gD1 antigen in a squalene/water formulation in guinea pigs (87,88). Antibody titers 4.4-fold higher than those generated by gD2 bound to alum were achieved with the low-oil o/w emulsion, compared to 7.7-fold higher titers elicited with CFA. Animals vaccinated with either the o/w or CFA formulations had a high level of protection against primary HSV2 disease (>90% protection) following viral challenge (87). Vaccination with a recombinant HSV gD2 glycoprotein antigen and the MTP-PE/squalene o/w formulation provided protection from recurrent as well as primary HSV disease, indicating the potential for development of an effective HSV-2 vaccine (89).

It is clear that use of low-oil o/w emulsions as vehicles combined with muramyl peptides can elicit antibody titers in the range of those obtainable with high-oil w/o formulations while reducing the potential toxicities substantially.

Liposomes

Liposomes have an extensive history as adjuvant vehicles, as has been recently reviewed (90-93). Liposomes of two types are in common use as adjuvants. Multilamellar liposomes (1-10-μm diameter) vaccines are typically generated by addition of soluble antigen to lyophilized liposome preparations. Unilamellar vesicle vaccines (60-150-nm diameter) are easily formed by dialysis of detergent from phospholipid/detergent micelles in the presence of antigen.

Liposomes have been employed as vehicles to carry additional adjuvants such as muramyl dipeptide or lipid A as well as antigen. Multilamellar liposomes (MLV) have been used to entrap hepatitis B surface antigen (HBsAg) or HBsAg plus assorted immunostimulators, including MDP (94). Subcutaneous administration of liposomes containing HBsAg to guinea pigs enhanced titers about fivefold over those achieved with free surface antigen. Addition of MDP to the liposomes enhanced the antibody production to 12-fold compared to free HBsAg. This enhancement was comparable to that achieved with alum. Only by mixing HBsAg with liposomes and B pertussis was a response greater than that of alum achieved.

Antibody responses to MLV liposomes can be increased by the incorporation of hydrophobic derivatives of muramyl peptides into the bilayer. MTP-PE employed with entrapped HSV glycoprotein gD2 in MLV elicited antibody titers in guinea pigs twofold higher than antigen bound to alum, but only 32% of those obtained with CFA and 50% of those achieved with a low-oil emulsion adjuvant (88). MTP-PE was added to MLV containing an acylated 23aa peptide from herpes simplex gD1 (95). The acylation of peptides facilitates their display on the surface of the liposome vesicle. The antibody response to the liposome-associated peptide was 10-fold greater than for free peptide and comparable to that achieved with peptide plus CFA. This response was increased to 40-fold over free peptide upon the addition of soluble MDP and 80-fold with MTP-PE. The addition of detoxified lipid A (MPL) generated titers similar to those achieved with MTP-PE, whereas the combination of MTP-PE and MPL resulted in a 160-fold stimulation (73). The detection of CMI, as measured by lymphoproliferation, required both liposome presentation and the inclusion of muramyl peptide. A similar system using cholera toxin associated with membrane-bound ganglioside GM1 gave about a fivefold increase in humoral antibody associated with liposome display compared to free cholera toxin (96). This enhanced immunogenicity was increased to 11-fold with the inclusion of the lipophilic muramyl peptide L18 MDP, to 50-fold with B30-MDP, and to 162-fold with lipid A. A similar result was reported in which 6-O stearyl MDP was less effective at boosting humoral responses to a hydrophobic DNP tripeptide associated with MLV vesicles than was lipid A (97).

A related effort has utilized a variety of lipophilic MDPs (with emphasis on the branched chain 6-O acyl derivatives B30 and B48) with unilamellar vesicles (86,98). Association of influenza hemagglutinin with unilamellar vesicles (virosomes) had previously been shown to increase antibody titers to influenza hemagglutinin by 5-10-fold over those achieved with protein micelles (99,100). Comparisons of the antibody titers obtained with a wide variety of MDP derivatives and influenza hemagglutinin in four vehicles (Freund's-like high oil, Ribi-like low oil, liposomes, and phosphate-buffered saline (PBS) showed that the two long branched-chain acyl derivatives (B30-MDP and B48-MDP) had superior efficacy/pyrogenicity ratios to hydrophobic straight-chain derivatives (101). The use of B30-MDP with influenza hemagglutinin resulted in a 30-fold increase in antibody compared to protein in saline. The inclusion of B30-MDP in liposomes resulted in a 1.5-fold increase in antibody titer over B30-MDP in PBS. The addition of B30-MDP to Freund's-type oil or Ribi-type oil emulsions gave 2-2.5-fold increases. The magnitude of the DTH response was similar for all four vehicles. The fact that the liposome and emulsion vehicles did not dramatically enhance immunogenicity compared to PBS may be due to the formation of an unusually immunoactive B30-MDP ovalbumin complex in PBS. B30-MDP has also been added to liposomes containing hepatitis B surface antigen; however, the substitution of detoxified lipid A derivatives for muramyl peptide appears to be more promising, particularly in booster applications (101).

In summary, the use of liposomes in combination with muramyl peptides (or further combinations with detoxified lipid A or trehalose dimycolate) boosts primary and, in some cases, secondary humoral responses many-fold over those observed with antigen in saline or antigen bound to alum. Cellular responses measured by T-cell proliferation or delayed hypersensitivity (DTH) are generated with all the muramyl peptide liposome systems. In addition, the potential for the generation of cytotoxic lymphocytes by the use of fusogenic liposomes capable of cytoplasmic antigen delivery remains an inviting possibility (102,103).

Covalent Conjugates

Muramyl dipeptides have been shown to elicit antibodies to numerous synthetic peptide antigens after conjugation to a carrier, including diphtheria toxin, streptococcal M-type 24 protein, foot-and-mouth disease virus, *Plasmodium* circumsporozoite protein, and hepatitis B surface antigen (104). Responses are further enhanced by direct conjugation of the MDP derivative to the peptide-toxoid conjugate, and the ratios of peptide to toxoid antibodies may increase dramatically. These tripartite conjugates are often delivered in saline.

Conjugates of the beta subunit of human chorionic gonadotropin with muramyl dipeptide or murabutide administered bound to alum induced a higher antibeta hCG response in mice than a beta-hCG-tetanus toxoid conjugate given with alum. These antibodies were capable of neutralizing hCG activity in vivo (105). A conjugate of influenza hemagglutinin peptide-tetanus toxoid covalently linked to MDP was capable of substituting for CFA for the induction of protection against an in vivo viral challenge infection, whereas the administration of free MDP in a mixture with the peptide-TT conjugate failed to afford significant protection (106). Likewise, coupling of a muramyl tripeptide to pneumococcal polysaccharide type 3 enhanced the immunogenicity of PS (107). In contrast to these reports, we observed that HSV gD2 protein covalently linked to nor-MDP was significantly less immunogenic in guinea pigs than gD2 combined with MDP in a low-oil emulsion, as measured by antibody titer, and afforded poorer protection against a viral challenge (87). Presumably this difference was due to the ratio of MDP to protein in the two cases; the covalent conjugate vaccine delivered 1000-fold less MDP per dose. Thus, covalent conjugation of MDP appears to be useful for peptide epitopes where a higher dose of the epitope is delivered in each vaccine compared to whole-protein antigens.

SPECIES VARIATION IN VEHICLE REQUIREMENTS FOR MURAMYL PEPTIDE AND ANTIGEN DELIVERY

Our own research has indicated that the vehicle used to deliver the muramyl peptide/antigen mixture is of uppermost importance and that large species differences exist in the requirement of vehicle for maximal immune response. We have concentrated on the lipophilic muramyl tripeptide MTP-PE in these studies, but very similar results have been obtained with other muramyl peptide derivatives. MTP-PE and antigen have been delivered in a variety of vehicles, including saline and various low-percentage metabolizable oil formulations. We have used squalene with oil concentrations of 5% or less to minimize side effects encountered with nonmetabolizable oils or high oil concentrations. Two basic types of oil formulations have been used: large droplet (1-10 μm), low-stability emulsions made with low-pressure devices (<1000 psi), such as a syringe and needle, and highly stable, small-droplet emulsions (200-500 nm) made in a high-pressure device ($\sim 10,000$ psi), such as the Microfluidizer. Using these formulations, we have discovered that small animals (rodents) respond equivalently to antigen and MTP-PE presented in both types of formulations, whereas large animals (goats and primates) require stable, small-droplet emulsion vehicles to achieve maximal immune responses. These results are consistent in experiments using a wide variety of antigens, including influenza, herpes simplex, and human immunodeficiency virus glycoproteins and malaria circumsporozoite proteins. The following examples with herpes simplex glycoprotein D and influenza vaccine illustrate this point.

Response of Guinea Pigs and Baboons to HSV gD2

The critical role of the vehicle or carrier formulation in evoking an immune response to a soluble antigen when combined with a muramyl dipeptide is demonstrated by analysis of the antibody response of baboons immunized with HSV glycoprotein gD2 presented in various vaccine formulations as shown in Table 1. The vehicles tested included alum, MTP-PE

Table 1 HSV Vaccine Trial 1 in Baboons[a]

Group	N	Adjuvant[b]		gD2 dose (μg)	gD2 ELISA titer[c]			CMI[d]
		Name	Dose (μg)		Bleed 1_3	Bleed 2_3	Bleed 3_3	
1	4	MTP-PE/LO	50	25	140 ± 63	788 ± 331	1320 ± 430	ND
2	4	MTP-PE/LO	1000	25	91 ± 70	1097 ± 565	3883 ± 2401	ND
3	4	Alum	400	25	1075 ± 785	880 ± 343	1993 ± 1156	1/4
4	4	MTP-PE/IFA	250	25	24101 ± 5423	62775 ± 28634	250382 ± 64771	4/4
5	4	IFA	250	25	2591 ± 2280	7631 ± 6563	66132 ± 75095	3/4
6	4	MTP-PE	250	25	31 ± 14	257 ± 91	833 ± 446	1/4

[a]Animals were immunized three times at 3-week intervals by intramuscular inoculation with the indicated vaccine.

[b]MTP-PE/LO = 4% squalene, 0.008% Tween-80, PBS plus MTP-PE at the indicated dose.

[c]ELISA titers expressed as geometric mean ± standard error of the mean measured 3 weeks following each immunization.

[d]Cellular mediated immunity measured as fraction of animals showing a positive lymphoproliferative response to gD2 antigen defined as a stimulation index of 3 or greater for bleed 3_3.

in a low-oil emulsion formulation, IFA, MTP-PE plus antigen emulsi-fied in IFA, and MTP-PE alone. Animals immunized with gD2 adsorbed to alum had a GMT of 1993 following the third immunization. In aqueous solution, MTP-PE spontaneously forms micelles of <10-nm diameter due to its amphipathic character. Animals immunized with gD2 combined with these MTP-PE micelles had a GMT only 40% that of the recipients of the alum-bound vaccine. Likewise, animals immunized with gD2 com-bined with MTP-PE delivered in a low-oil emulsion of limited stability (MTP-PE/LO) had low antibody titers comparable to those elicited with alum (GMT 1320 with 50 μg MTP-PE and 3883 with 1000 μg MTP-PE). In contrast, the presentation of gD2 combined with MTP-PE in an IFA emulsion generated a GMT of 250,000 compared to gD2 with IFA alone with a GMT of 66,132. Paralleling the antibody titers, lymphoprolifera-tive responses were readily detected for animals immunized with gD2 com-bined with MTP-PE in IFA or with IFA alone but were infrequent for alum or MTP-PE micelle vehicles. This dramatic enhancement of the adjuvant potency of MTP-PE by IFA could have been due to the high oil concentration or the physical properties of the emulsion, or both.

A second experiment, also performed in baboons, demonstrates more clearly the role of the physical characteristics of emulsion itself. As shown in Table 2, baboons were immunized with gD2 bound to alum or com-bined with low-oil formulations MF1 or MF59. For the MF1 formula-tion, MTP-PE was used as the sole emulsifying agent, whereas for MF59 the polyoxyethylene sorbitan ester detergents Tween-80 and Span 85 were used as the emulsifying agents. MF1 is a stable emulsion alone but is de-stabilized upon addition of saline or gD2 antigen, presumably due in part to charge neutralization of the oil droplet surface. In comparison, the MF59 emulsion is stable upon addition of the gD2 antigen. Baboons im-munized with gD2 bound to alum had GMT of 3821, and those receiving gD2 with MTP-PE/MF1 had a comparable GMT of 5295. The group im-munized with the stable emulsion formulation, gD2 with MTP-PE/MF59, had a four- to fivefold higher titer of 24,263.

In contrast to baboons, guinea pigs are insensitive to the physical characteristics of the vehicle formulation. As shown in Figure 1, guinea pigs immunized with 12 μg of gD2 combined with MTP-PE/LO or with MTP-PE/MF59 had indistinguishable antibody responses and were equally well protected from clinically apparent lesions following challenge with HSV-2 (Figure 2). For both vehicles, five of eight animals developed clini-cally apparent lesions, with total average lesion scores of 0.24 and 0.26 for MF59 and LO for the 14-day acute disease phase observation period;

Table 2   HSV Vaccine Trial 2 in Baboons[a]

Group	N	Adjuvant[b] Dose (µg)	Adjuvant[b] Name	gD2 dose (µg)	gD2 ELISA titer[c] Bleed 1_1	Bleed 1_3	Bleed 2_1	Bleed 2_3	Bleed 3_1	Bleed 3_3
1	3	400	Alum	25	635 ± 244	1337 ± 244	3092 ± 456	3844 ± 264	4902 ± 363	3821 ± 794
2	3	100	MTP-PE/MF1	25	337 ± 258	800 ± 286	5900 ± 2520	6115 ± 2229	17848 ± 1400	5295 ± 1116
5	3	100	MTP-PE/MF59	25	1655 ± 1183	3776 ± 1749	12690 ± 4854	20912 ± 4724	25953 ± 9327	24263 ± 5150[d]

[a]Animals were immunized three times at 3-week intervals with the indicated vaccine administered by intramuscular administration.

[b]MTP-PE/MF1 = 1.6% squalene, 0.4 mg/ml MTP-PE mixed 1:1 (v/v) with antigen in phosphate buffer. MTP-PE/MF59 = 5% squalene, 0.5% Tween-80, 0.5% Span 85, 0.4 mg/ml MTP-PE mixed 1:1 (v/v) with antigen in phosphate buffer.

[c]ELISA titer expressed as geometric mean ± standard error of the mean. The timing of blood collection is indicated as number of weeks following each immunization; e.g., 2_1 is 1 week following the second immunization.

[d]N = 2; one animal died from causes not related to vaccination.

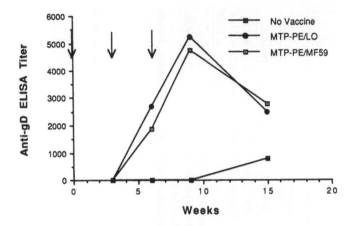

Figure 1 gD2 antibody titers in guinea pigs immunized with HSV gD2 in low-oil emulsion vaccine formulations. Groups of eight guinea pigs were immunized three times at 3-week intervals with 12 μg gD2 in the indicated vehicle by intramuscular administration. At week 12 they were infected by intravaginal instillation of 1.8×10^5 pfu of HSV-2. Geometric mean ELISA titers to gD2 are plotted for each bleed.

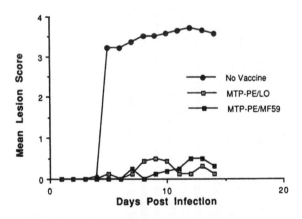

Figure 2 Protection of guinea pigs from HSV disease with gD2 in low-oil emulsion vaccine formulations. The clinical disease profile of immunized and control, unimmunized guinea pigs infected with HSV-2 as noted in Figure 1. Disease was measured on a scale of 0 (corresponding to no lesions) to 4 (corresponding to virtually confluent lesions covering the genital skin) (87).

no animals died. Both of these groups were well protected from the severe HSV challenge compared to the control group, in which seven of seven animals were infected, four of seven animals died, and the mean lesion score was 2.48. Mice are similar to guinea pigs in their nonresponsiveness to the vehicle formulation. Others have similarly reported that there was no difference in the immune response of guinea pigs immunized with a stable versus an unstable oil emulsion containing the adjuvant threonyl-MDP (108).

Response of Goats to Influenza Vaccine

The response of goats to influenza vaccine combined with MTP-PE in a variety of vehicles was determined. Animals received 15 μg of each hemagglutinin in a trivalent vaccine presented in saline alone, or combined with 200 μg of MTP-PE in the low-oil emulsions MTP-PE/LO, MF101, or MF59. The MF59 emulsion is similar in droplet size and stability to MF101 alone but shows improved stability compared to MF101 after mixing with influenza vaccine. The results of this experiment are illustrated in Figure 3. The vaccine alone gave low antibody titers (mean titer of 8 after one immunization and 7 after two immunizations). The MTP-PE/LO formulation gave improved but still low titers in the goats (mean titers of 55 and 524 following one and two immunizations). Titers were similar using the MF101 formulation (mean titer of 258 after one immunization and 858 after two immunizations) and were much higher with the MF59 formulation (884 and 3704 following one and two immunizations, respectively). Based on these results, it is apparent that goats, like baboons, require an emulsion of high stability to develop a good antibody response.

These examples illustrate the differences in response of small versus large animals to vaccines delivered with muramyl peptide in oil vehicles. These results appear to be consistent for a variety of animals with several different antigens. Small animals such as mice, hamsters, guinea pigs, and rabbits are able to make good antibody responses to antigens delivered with muramyl peptides in unstable oil emulsions, while species such as goats, baboons, rhesus monkeys, and chimpanzees require small-diameter, stable oil vehicles for effective antibody responses. The source of the difference in the sensitivity of large versus small animals to the faccine vehicle remains to be elucidated. Probable explanations may include species variation in intrinsic sensitivity to MDP or differences in the distribution of the vaccine between the site of immunization and the draining lymph node. Our belief is that humans will fit the large-animal model

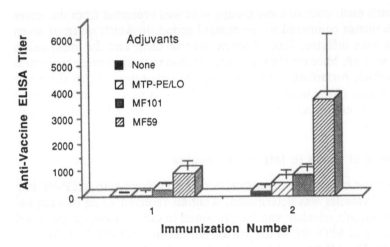

Figure 3 Adjuvant activity in goats with influenza vaccine. Groups of five animals each were immunized with 45 μg of hemagglutinin in a trivalent vaccine (15 μg each of hemagglutinin from H1N1, H3N2, and B strains), either alone or combined with 200 μg of MTP-PE in the MTP-PE/LO, MF101, or MF59 formulations. Animals were immunized intramuscularly three times at 3-week intervals, and antibody titers against the influenza vaccine were determined 14 days after each immunization. Plotted values represent geometric means and error bars represent standard errors for the groups.

and will require stable oil vehicles for effective antigen/adjuvant delivery. Our data indicate that using small-animal models for testing oil-based adjuvants can be misleading and that large-animal models should be used to verify the performance of formulations selected in small-animal systems.

Use of Muramyl Peptide Vaccine Adjuvants in Humans

Three vaccine trials using muramyl peptide-based adjuvants have been performed in humans to date. These include a trial using tetanus toxoid combined with Murabutide (109), human chorionic gonadotropin (hCG) peptide combined with nor-MDP (110), and a recombinant HIV envelope protein combined with MTP-PE (111). In the tetanus-Murabutide trial, patients were immunized with standard doses of tetanus toxoid combined with Murabutide doses ranging from 1.6 to 6.2 mg in saline. Although the combination of tetanus toxoid and Murabutide was safe, it provided only small, statistically insignificant increases in immune responses over tetanus toxoid alone. The vaccine used in the hCG trial was more complex and consisted of a synthetic peptide corresponding to an immunogenic region of hCG conjugated to a diphtheria toxoid carrier and mixed with nor-MDP in a 50:50 water-in-oil emulsion vehicle. The oil phase of the vehicle consisted of 80% squalene and 20% Arlacel A. Patients were divided into five groups that received graded doses of antigen and adjuvant from 50 μg of peptide-carrier plus 25 μg of MDP to 1000 μg of peptide-carrier plus 500 μg of MDP. Again the vaccine was safe, with transient myalgia being the only significant side effect. Antibody responses in this study were generally good, although no controls without adjuvant were included. The authors noted that the delivery vehicle was in some cases unstable, and that instability was associated with a subsequent lack of immunogenicity and increased side effects. In the HIV trial, patients were immunized with either 50 or 250 μg of a recombinant HIV envelope protein produced in yeast combined with 100 μg of MTP-PE and a vehicle consisting of 4% squalene and 0.008% Tween-80 (MTP-PE/LO). As in the other two studies, this vaccine was well tolerated, with minor pain at the injection site being the only significant side effect noted. Antibody responses to the vaccine were detectable but low, and measurable T-cell (lymphoproliferative) responses were generated. The emulsion vehicle used in this study was unstable and probably contributed to the low antibody responses detected.

These three trials all indicate that muramyl peptide adjuvanted vaccines can be safe in humans. The results of all three trials also stress that vehicles for vaccine delivery are important and that improved vehicles are necessary for generating good immune responses. The tetanus toxoid vaccine employed no vehicle and resulted in poor antibody responses even with very high muramyl peptide doses (6.2 mg). It should be noted that all study subjects had received prior immunizations with tetanus toxoid. Thus, the antibody response elicited was amnestic rather than primary. The relative utility or importance of adjuvant in these two cases is not clear. The hCG vaccine used a water-in-oil vehicle, but this vehicle was occasionally unstable. The instability of certain batches of the vehicle was directly related to poor antibody responses in patients. The HIV trial also employed an unstable vehicle and generated poor antibody responses. Our animal studies would imply that all three of the muramyl peptide/ vaccine combinations used in these studies could have been more effective if they were delivered in improved vehicles.

SUMMARY

It is clear that vaccines incorporating one of several different muramyl peptide derivatives can enhance both cellular and humoral response to a variety of antigens when formulated with an effective vehicle. Both liposomes and oil-in-water emulsions have been shown to potentiate immunogenicity in small rodent species when combined with muramyl peptides. Demonstration of the efficacy and safety of muramyl peptide formulations in primates is ongoing and appears to be promising when vehicle formulations are optimized.

A number of points related to the use of muramyl peptide formulations as vaccines remain to be addressed. These include determining the method of uptake of MDP by macrophages and lymphocytes and the mechanism of signal transduction for MDP-mediated activation. The synergistic effects of MDP with lipid A or trehalose dimycolate should be dissected to obtain increased immunogenicity without increased toxicity.

A continued study of vehicle formulation is equally important. The ability to target delivery of antigen, muramyl peptide, and other adjuvants to immunoactive cells remains critical. The ability of these formulations to establish memory and sustained immune responses needs to be investigated. Finally, the development of predictive in vitro assays for adjuvant efficacy and the establishment of a firm link between results in animal models and humans could minimize the number of animal experiments and dramatically accelerate the pace of formulation research.

ACKNOWLEDGMENTS

We would like to acknowledge the support of the Biocine Company; Dr. Dino Dina, for his continuing encouragement; Dr. D. Rick Lee, for help with the baboon immunizations; and Peter Anderson, for help with manuscript preparation. The order of authorship was determined by the drawing of lots.

REFERENCES

1. Freund J. The mode of action of immunologic adjuvants. Adv Tuberc Res 1956; 7:130.
2. Raffel S, Arnaud LE, Dukes DE, Huang JS. The role of the "wax" of the tubercle bacillis in establishing delayed hypersensitivity. II. Hypersensitivity to a protein antigen, egg albumin. J Exp Med 1949; 90:53.

3. White RG, Bernstock L, Johns RL, Lederer E. The influence of components of *M. tuberculosis* and other mycobacteria upon antibody production to ovalbumin. Immunology 1958; 1:54.

4. White RG, Jolles P, Samour D, Lederer E. Correlation of adjuvant activity and chemical structure of wax D fractions of mycobacteria. Immunology 1964; 7(24):158.

5. Adam A, Ciourbaru R, Petit JF, Lederer E. Isolation and properties of a macromolecular, water soluble, immunoadjuvant fraction from the cell wall of *Mycobacterium smegmatis*. Proc Natl Acad Sci USA 1972; 69:855.

6. Migliorie-Samour D, Jolles P. A hydrosoluble, adjuvant active mycobacterial "polysaccharide peptidoglycan glycan." Preparation by a simple extraction technique of the bacterial strains (strain peurois). FEBS Lett 1972; 25:301.

7. Hiu IJ. Water soluble and lipid free fraction from BCG with adjuvant and antitumor activity. Nature New Biol 1972; 238:241.

8. Ellouz F, Adam A, Ciourbaru R, Lederer E. Minimal structure requirements for adjuvant activity of bacterial peptidoglycan derivatives. Biochem Biophys Res Comm 1974; 590:1317.

9. Merser C, Sinay P, Adam A. Total synthesis and adjuvant activity of bacterial peptidoglycan derivatives. Biochem Biophys Res Com 1975; 66:1316.

10. Kotani S, Watanabe Y, Kinoshita F, Shimono T, Morisaki I, Shiba T, Kusumoto S, Tarumi Y, Ikenaka K. Immunoadjuvant activities of synthetic N-acetylmuramyl peptides or amino acids. Biken J 1975; 18:105.

11. Fevrier M, Birrien JL, Leclerc C, Chedid L, Liaco-Poulos P. The macrophage is the target cell of the synthetic adjuvant muramyl dipeptide. Eur J Immunol 1978; 8:558.

12. Tanaka A, Nagao S, Saito R, Kotani S, Kusumoto S, Shiba T.Correlation of stereochemically specific structure in muramyl dipeptide between macrophage activation and adjuvant activity. Biochem Biophys Res Commun 1977; 77:621.

13. Tanaka A, Tsujimoto M, Kato K, Kotani S, Kusumoto S, Inage M, Shiba T, Yano I, Kawata S, Yogogawa K. Macrophage activation by bacterial cell walls and related synthetic compounds. Infect Immunol 1979; 25:48.

14. Waters RV, Ferraresi RW. Muramyldipeptide stimulation of particle clearance in several animal species. J Reticuloendothel Soc 1980; 28:457.

15. Fraser-Smith EB, Waters RV, Matthews TR. Correlation between *in vivo* anti-pseudomonas and anti-candida activities and clearance of carbon by the res for various muramyldipeptide analogues using normal and immunosuppressed mice. Infect Immunol 1982; 35:105.

16. Cummings NP, Pabst MJ, Johnson Jr, RB. Activation of macrophages for enhanced release of superoxide anion and greater killing of candida albicans by injected muramyl dipeptide. J Exp Med 1980; 152:1659.

17. Pabst MJ, Johnson Jr, RB. Increased production of superoxide anion by macrophages exposed *in vitro* to muramyl dipeptide or lipopolysaccharide. J Exp Med 1980; 151:101.

18. Whal SM, Whal LM, McCarthy JB, Chedid L, Mergenhagen SE. Macrophage activation by mycobacterial water soluble compounds and synthetic muramly dipeptide. J Immunol 1979; 122:2226.

19. Juy D, Chedid L. Comparison between macrophage activation and enhancement of non-specific resistance to tumors by mycobacterial immunoadjuvants. Proc Natl Acad Sci USA 1975; 72:4105.

20. Fidler IJ, Sone S, Fogler WF, Barnes ZL. Eradication of spontaneous metastasis and activation of alveolar macrophages by intravenous injection of liposomes containing muramyl dipeptide. Proc Natl Acad Sci USA 1981; 78: 1680.

21. Fidler IJ, Sone S, Fogler WE, Smith D, Braun DG, Tarcsay L, Gisler RH, Schroit AJ. Efficacy of liposomes containing a lipophilic muramyl dipeptide derivative for activating the tumoricidal properties of alveolar macrophages *in vivo*. J Biol Response Modif 1982; 1:43.

22. Oppenheim JJ, Togawa A, Chedid L, Mizel S. Components of mycobacteria and muramyl dipeptide with adjuvant activity induce lymphocyte activating factor. Cell Immunol 1980; 50:71.

23. Parant M, Vimit M-A, Damais D, Riveau G, Chedid L. Production of differentiation-stimulating factor for murine leukemic myeloblast line by monocytic cells stimulated by a non-pyrogenic muramyl dipeptide derivative. Exp Hematol NY 1985; 221.

24. Saiki I, Saito S, Fujita C, Ishida H, Iida J, Murata J, Hasegawa A, Azuma I. Induction of tumoricidal macrophages and production of cytokines by synthetic muramyl dipeptide analogues. Vaccine 1988; 6:238.

25. Bahr GM, Chedid LA, Behbhani K. Induction *in vivo* and *in vitro* of macrophage membrane interleukin-1 by adjuvant active synthetic muramyl peptides. Cell Immunol 1987; 107:443.

26. Parant M, Parant F, Vinit M-A, Jupin C, Noso Y, Chedid L. Priming effect of muramyl peptides for induction by lipopolysaccharides of tumor necrosis factor production in mice. J Leukocyte Biol 1990; 47:164.

27. Fuks BB, Rakhmilevich AL, Pimenov AA, Dubrovskaya AC. *In vitro* and *in vivo* activation of tumor necrosis factor production by the combination of lipopolysaccharide and muramyl dipeptide. Byull EKSP Biol Med 1987; 104: 497.

28. Akahane K, Yamaguchi F, Kita Y, Une T, Osada Y. Stimulation of macrophages by muroctasin to produce colony-stimulating factors. Arzneim-Forsch 1990; 40:179.

29. Galelli A, Charlot B, Phillips NC, Chedid L. Induction of colony-stimulating activity in mice by injection of liposomes containing lipophilic muramyl peptide derivatives. Cancer Res 1989; 49:810.

30. Yamaguchi F, Akasuki Y, Tsukada W. Induction of colony-stimulating factor and stimulation of stem cell proliferation by injection of muroctasin. Arzneim-Forsch 1988; 38:980.

31. Sanceau J, Falcott R, Beranger F, Carter DB, Wietzerbin J. Secretion of interleukin-6 by human monocytes stimulated by muramyl dipeptide and tumor necrosis factor alpha. Immunology 1990; 69:52.

32. Wachsmuth ED. Stimulation of cell proliferation in rabbits by MTP-PE, a lipophilic muramyl peptide. Virchows Arch B Cell Pathol Incl Mol Pathol 1988; 54:195.

33. Wachsmuth EO, Huber J. Stimulant effect of the immunomodulator MTP-PE on monocytic cells in the guinea pig. Virchows Arch B Cell Pathol Incl Mol Pathol 1989; 58:450.

34. Wuest B, Wachsmuth ED. Stimulatory effect of N-acetylmuramyl dipeptide *in vivo* on proliferation of bone marrow progenitor cells in mice. Infect Immunol 1982; 37:452.

35. Souvannavong V, Brown S, Adam A. The synthetic immunomodulator muramyl dipeptide (MDP) can stimulate activated B cells. Mol Immunol 1988; 25:385.

36. Souvannavong V, Brown S, Adam A. Muramyl dipeptide (MDP) synergizes with interleukin 2 and interleukin 4 to stimulate respectively the differentiation and proliferation of B cells. Cell Immunol 1990; 126:106.

37. Souvannavong V, Adam A. Restoration and stimulation of the *in vitro* immune response of B cells to sheep erythrocytes by interleukins and muramyl dipeptide. Biochem Biophys Res Commun 1984; 125:431.

38. Souvannavong V, Rimsky Z, Adam A. *In vitro* immune response to sheep erythrocytes in macrophage depleted cultures restored with interleukin 1 or a monokine from resident macrophages and stimulation by an N-acetylmuramyl-L-alanyl-D-isoglutamine. Biochem Biophys Res Commun 1983; 114: 721.

39. Gisler RH, Dietrich FM, Baschang G, Brownhill A, Schumann G, Staber FG, Tarcsay L, Wachsmuth ED, Dakor P. New developments in drugs enhancing the immune response: activation of lymphocytes and accessory cells by muramyl-dipeptides. In: Turk JL, Park D, eds. Drugs and Immune Response. London: Macmillan, 1979:133.

40. Kishter S, Hoffman FA, Pizza PA. Production and response to interleukin 2 by cultured T cells. Effects of lithium chloride and other putative modulators. J Biol Response Modif 1985; 4:185.

41. Leclerc C, Bourgeois E, Chedid L. Demonstration of muramyl dipeptide induced T suppressor cells responsible for muramyl dipeptide immunosuppressive activity. Eur J Immunol 1982; 12:249.

42. Audibert F, Chedid L, Lefrancier P, Choay J. Distinctive adjuvanticity of synthetic analogs of mycobacterial water soluble components. Cell Immunol 1976; 21:243.

43. Sharma SD, Tsai U, Krahenbul JL, Remington JS. Augmentation of mouse natural killer cell activity by muramyl dipeptide and its analogues. Cell Immunol 1981; 62:101.

44. Talmadge JE, Schneider M, Collins M, Phillips H. Augmentation of natural killer cell activity in tissue by liposomes incorporating muramyl tripeptides. J Immunol 1985; 135:1477.

45. Osada Y, Otani T, Sato M, Une T, Matsumoto K, Ogawa H. Polymorphonuclear leukocyte activation by a synthetic muramyl dipeptide analog. Infect Immunol 1982; 38:848.

46. Dietrich FM, Hochkeppel HK, Lukas B. Enhancement of host resistance against virus infections by MTP-PE, a synthetic, lipophilic muramyl peptide. I. Increased survival in mice and guinea pigs after single drug administration prior to infection and the effect of MTP-PE on interferon levels in sera and lungs. Int J Immunopharmacol 1986; 8:931.

47. Fogler WE, Fidler IJ. Modulation of the immune response by muramyl dipeptide. In: Immune Modulation Agents and Their Mechanisms. Chirigos M, Fenichel R, eds. New York: Marcel Dekker, 1984:499.

48. Koff WC, Showalter SD, Hampar B, Fidler IJ. Protection of mice against fatal herpes simplex type 2 liposomes containing muramyl tripeptide. Science 1985; 228:495.

49. Krahenbuhl JL, Humphres RC. Effects of treatment with muramyl dipeptide on resistance to mycobacterium leprae and mycobacterium marinum infection in mice. Immunopharmacology 1983; 5:329.

50. Kotani S, Watenabe Y, Shimono T, Horada K, Shiba T, Kusomoto S, Yokogawa K, Taniguchi M. Correlation between the immunoadjuvant activities and pyrogenicities of synthetic acetylmuramyl peptides or N-acetyl muramyl amino acids. Biken J 1976; 19:9.

51. Dinarello C, Elin RJ, Chedid L, Wolff SM. The pyrogenicity of synthetic muramyldipeptide and two structural analogues. J Infect Dis 1978; 138:760.

52. Riveau G, Hosmalin A, Cavelli C, Lefrancier P, Chedid L. Decrease in pyrogenicity of muramyl dipeptide after coupling with LHRH. J Leukocyte Biol 1988; 44:448.

53. Chedid L, Parant MA, Audibert FM, Riveau GJ, Parant FJ, Lederer E, Choay JP, Lefrancier PL. Biological activity of a new synthetic muramyl peptide adjuvant devoid of pyrogenicity. Infect Immunol 1982; 35:417.

54. Allison AC, Byars NE, Waters RV. Immunological adjuvants: efficacy and safety considerations. In: Nervig RM, Gough PM, Kaeberle ML, Whatstore CA, eds. Advances in Carriers and Adjuvants for Veterinary Biologics. Ames, IA: Iowa State University Press, 1986:91.

55. Tsujimoto M, Kotani S, Kinoshita F, Karoh S, Shiba T, Kusumoto S. Adjuvant activity of 6-O-Acyl-Muramyldipeptides to enhance primary cellular and humoral immune responses in guinea pigs: Adaptability to various vehicles and pyrogenicity. Infect Immunol 1986; 53:511.

56. Gisler RH, Shumann G, Sackmann W, Pericin C, Tarscay L, Deitrich FM. A novel muramyl peptide, MTP-PE: profile of biological activities. In: Yamamura Y, Kotani S, eds. Immunomodulation by Microbial Products and Related Synthetic Compounds. Amsterdam: Excerpta Medica, 1982:167.

57. Emori K, Anotaraka A. Granuloma formation by synthetic bacterial cell wall fragment: Muramyl dipeptide. Infect Immunol 1978; 19:613.
58. Tanaka A, Emori K. Epithiloid granuloma formation by a synthetic bacterial cell wall component, muramyl dipeptide (MDP). Am J Pathol 1980; 98:733.
59. Emori K, Nagao S, Shigematsu N, Kotari S, Tsujimoto M, Shiba T, Kusumoto S, Tanaka A. Granuloma formation by muramyl peptide associated with branched fatty acids, a structure probably essential for tubercle formation by Mycobacterian tuberculosis. Infect Immunol 1985; 49:244.
60. Zidek Z, Masek K, Jiricka A. Arthritogenic activity of synthetic immunoadjuvant muramyl dipeptide. Infect Immunol 1982; 35:674.
61. Nagao S, Tanaka A. Muramyl peptide-induced adjuvant arthritis. Infect Immunol 1980; 28:624.
62. Chang, YH, Pearson CM, Chedid L. Adjuvant polyarthritis. V. Induction by N-acetylmuramyl-L-alanyl-D-isoglutamide, the smallest peptide of bacterial peptidoglycan. J Exp Med 1981; 153:1021.
63. Koga T, Kakimoto K, Horifuji T, Kotari S, Sumiyoshi A, Saisho K. Muramyl dipeptide induces acute joint inflammation in the mouse. Microbiol Immunol 1986; 30:717.
64. Kohashi O, Tunaka A, Kotani S, Shiba T, Kusamato S, Yokogawa K, Kawata S, Ozawa A. Arthritis inducting ability of a synthetic adjuvant N-acetylmuramylpeptides and bacterial disaccharide peptides related to different oil vehicles and their composition. Infect Immunol 1980; 29:70.
65. Fox A, Hammer ME, Lill P, Burch TG, Barrish G. Experimental uveitis elicited by peptideglycan-polysaccharide complexes, lipopolysaccharide, and muramyl dipeptide. Arch Ophthalmol 1984; 102:1063.
66. Waters R, Terrell TG, Jones CH. Uveitis induction in the rabbit by muramyl dipeptides. Infect Immunol 1986; 51:816.
67. Ribi EE, Cantrell JL, Von Escher KB, Schwartzman SM. Enhancement of endotoxic shock by N-acetylmuramyl-L-alanyl-(L-seryl)-D-isoglutamine (muramyl dipeptide). Cancer Res 1979; 39:4756.
68. Takada H, Galanos G. Enhancement of endotoxin lethality and generation of anaphylactoid reactions by lipopolysaccharides in muramyl dipeptide-treated mice. Infect Immunol 1987; 55.
69. Nagao S, Tanaka A. Necrotic inflammatory reaction induced by muramyl dipeptide in guinea pigs sensitized by tubercle bacilli. J Exp Med 1985; 162:401.
70. Nagao S, Takada H, Yagawa K, Kutsukake H, Shiba T, Kusumoto S, Kawata S, Hasegawa A, Kiso M, Azuma I, Tanuka A, Kotani S. Structural requirements of muramylpeptides for induction of necrosis at sites primed with *Alycobacterium tuberculosis* in guinea pigs. Infect Immunol 1987; 55: 1279.
71. Audibert FM, Parant C, Damais C, Lefrancier P, Denien M, Choay J, Chedid L. Disassociation of immunostimulating activities of muramyldipeptide

(MDP) by linking amino acids or peptides to the glutaminyl residue. Biochem Biophys Res Commun 1980; 96:915.

72. Kotani S, Hinoshita F, Mousaki I, Shimono T, Okunaga T, Takada H, Tsiyimoto M, Watanabe Y, Koto K, Shiba T, Kusumoto S, Okada S. Immunoadjuvant activities of synthetic 6-O-acyl N acetyl muramyl L alanyl D isoglutamine with special reference to the effect of its administration with liposomes. Biken J 1977; 20:95.

73. Naylor PT, Larsen HS, Huang L, Rouse BT. In vivo induction of antiherpes simplex immune response by type 1 antigen and lipid A incorporated into liposomes. Infect Immunol 1982; 36:1209.

74. Davis S, Hadraft J, Palin K. Medical and pharmaceutical applications of emulsions. In: Becher P, ed. Encyclopedia of Emulsion Technology. Vol 2. New York: Marcel Dekker, 1985:159-238.

75. Brugh M, Stone H, Lipton H. Comparison of inactivated Newcastle disease viral vaccines containing different emulsion adjuvants. Am J Vet Res 1983; 44:72.

76. Reynolds J, Herrington D, Crabbs C, Peters C, DiLuzio N. Adjuvant activity of a novel metabolizable lipid emulsion with inactivated viral vaccines. Infect Immunol 1980; 28:937.

77. Ribi E, Takayama K, Milner K, Gray GR, Goren M, Parker R, McLaughlin C, Kelly M. Regression of tumors by an endotoxin combined with trehalose mycolates of differing structure. Cancer Immunol Immunother 1976; 1:265-270.

78. Retzinger G, Meredith S, Hunter R, Takayama K, Kezdy F. Identification of the physiologically active state of the mycobacterial glycolipid trehalose 6-6' dimiycolate and the role of fibrinogen in the biologic activities of trehalose 6-6' dimycolate monolayers. J Immunol 1982; 129:735.

79. Musiki KN, Lange W, Brehmer W, Ribi E. Immunologic activities of nontoxic lipid A: enhancement of non-specific resistance in combination with trehalose dimycolate against viral infection and adjuvant effects. Int J Immunopharmacol 1986; 8:339.

80. Woodward L. Adjuvant activity of water-insoluble surfactants. Lab Animal Sci 1989; 39(3):222.

81. Hunter R, Strickland F, Kezdy FJ. The adjuvant activity of nonionic block polymer surfactants. I. The role of hydrophile-lipophile balance. J Immunol 1981; 127:1244.

82. Hunter R, Bennett B. The adjuvant activity of nonionic block polymer surfactants. II. Antibody formation and inflammation related to the structure of triblock and octablock copolymers. J Immunol 1984; 133:3167.

83. Hunter R, Bennett B. The adjuvant activity of nonionic block polymer surfactants. III. Characterization of selected biologically active surfaces. Scand J Immunol 1986; 23:287.

84. Byars N, Allison A. Adjuvant formulation for use in vaccines to elicit both cell-mediated and humoral immunity. Vaccine 1987; 5:223.

85. Byars N, Allison A, Harmon M, Kendal A. Enhancements of antibody response to influenza B virus haemagglutinin by use of a new adjuvant formulation. Vaccine 1990; 8:49.

86. Tsujimoto M, Kotani S, Shiba T, Kusumoto S. Adjuvant activity of 6-O-Acyl-Muramyldipeptides to enhance primary cellular and humoral immune responses in guinea pigs: Dose-response and local reactions observed with selected compounds. Infect Immunol 1986; 53:517.

87. Sanchez-Pescador L, Burke R, Ott G, Van Nest G. The effect of adjuvants on the efficacy of a recombinant herpes simplex virus glycoprotein vaccine. J Immunol 1988; 141:1720.

88. Sanchez-Pescador L, Burke RL, Ott G, Ng P, Larsen C, Gervase B, Van Nest G. A comparison of adjuvant efficacy for a recombinant herpes simplex virus glycoprotein vaccine. In: Laskey L, Fox CF, eds. Technological Advances in Vaccine Development. New York: Academic Press, 1988:455.

89. Burke R, Van Nest G, Gervase B, Goldbeck C, Dina D, Brown P, Wheelwright, Ott G. Development of an HSV subunit vaccine: Effect of adjuvant composition and antigen dose. In: Meheus A, Spier RE, eds. Vaccines for Sexually Transmitted Disease, 1989:191.

90. Gregoriadis G. Immunological adjuvants: A role for liposomes. Immunol Today 1990; 11:89.

91. Rouse BT. Liposomes as carriers of antigens as wells as other molecules involved in immunity. J Am Vet Med Assoc 1982; 181:988.

92. van Rooijen N, van Nieuwmegen R, Kors N. Liposomes as immunological adjuvants. In: Cell Function and Differentiation. Part A. New York: Alan R Liss, 1982:281.

93. Alving CR. Liposomes as carriers for vaccines. In: Ostro M, ed. Liposomes from Biophysics to Therapeutics. New York: Marcel Dekker, 1987:195-218.

94. Gregoriadis G, Manesis EK. Liposomes as immunological adjuvants for hepatitis B surface antigens. In: Tom, Six H, eds. Liposomes and Immunology. New York: Elsevier-North Holland, 1980:271-283.

95. Brynestad K, Babbitt B, Huang L, Rouse BT. Influence of peptide acylation, liposome incorporation and synthetic immunomodulators on the immunogenicity of a 1-23 peptide of glycoprotein D of herpes simplex virus: implications for subunit vaccines. J Virol 1990; 64:680.

96. Alving CR, Richards RC, Moss J, Alving LI, Clemonts JD, Shiba T, Katuni S, Wirtz RA, Hockmeyer WT. Effectiveness of liposomes as potential carriers of vaccine: applications to cholera toxin and human malaria sporozoite antigen. Vaccine 1986; 4:166.

97. Zigterman G, Jansye M, Snippe H, Willers J. Immunomodulating properties of substances to be used in combinations with liposomes. Int Arch Appl Immunol 1986; 81:245.

98. Tsujimoto M, Kotani F, Kinoshita F, Kanoh S, Shiba T, Kusumoto S. Adjuvant activity of 6-O actl-muramyldipeptides to enhance primary cellular

and humoral immune responses in guinea pigs—adaptability to various vehicles and pyrogenicity. Infect Immunol 1986; 53:511.

99. Oxford JS, Hockley DJ, Heath TD, Patterson S. The interaction of influenza virus haemagglutinin with phospholipid vesicles: morphological and immunological studies. J Gen Virol 1981; 52:329.

100. Berezin VE, Zaides JM, Isawa ES, Actamanov AF, Zhacinoo VM. Controlled organization of multimolecular complexes of enveloped virus glycoproteins: study of immunogenicity. Vaccine 1988; 6:450.

101. Tsujimoto M, Kotani S, Okunaga T, Kubo T, Takada H, Kubo T, Shiba T, Kusumoto S, Takahashi T, Goto Y, Kinoshita F. Enhancement of humoral immune responses against viral vaccines by a non-pyrogenic 6-O-acylmuramyl peptide and synthetic low toxicity analogues of lipid A. Vaccine 1989; 7:39.

102. Straubinger R, Duzgunes N, Papahadjopoulos D. pH-Sensitive liposomes mediate cytoplasmic delivery of encapsulated macromolecules. FEBS Lett 1985; 179:148.

103. Connor J, Huang L. Efficient cytoplasmic delivery of a fluorescent dye by pH-sensitive liposomes. J Cell Biol 1985; 101:582.

104. Audibert F, Leclerc C, Chedid L. Muramyl peptides as immunopharmacological response modifiers. In: Torrance, Ed. Biological Response Modifiers. San Diego: Academic Press, 1986:307.

105. Schutze MP, Leclerc C, Jolivet M, Deriaud E, Audibert FA, Chang CC, Chedid L. A potential anti-pregnancy vaccine built by conjugation of the beta-subunit of human chorionic gonadotropin to adjuvant-active muramyl peptide. Am J Reprod Immunol Microbiol 1987; 14:18.

106. Shapira M, Jolivet M, Arnon R. A synthetic vaccine against influenza with built-in adjuvanticity. Int J Immunopharmacol 1985; 7:719.

107. Yin J-Z, Bell MK, Thorbecke GJ. Effect of various adjuvants on the antibody response of mice to pneumococcal polysaccharides. J Biol Response Modif 1989; 8:190.

108. Lidgate D, Fu R, Byars N, Foster L, Fleitman JS. Formulation of vaccine adjuvant muramyldipeptides. 3. Processing optimization characterization and bioactivity of an emulsion vehicle. Pharm Res 1989; 6:748.

109. Telzak E, Wolfe SM, Dinarello CA, Conlon T, Kholz AE, Bahr GM, Choag JP, Morin A, Chedid L. Clinical evaluation of the immunoadjuvant Murabutide, a derivative of MDP, administered with a tetanus toxoid vaccine. J Infect Dis 1986; 153:628.

110. Jones WR, Judd SJ, Ing RMY, Powell J, Bradley J, Denholm EH, Mueller UW, Griffin PD, Stevens VC. Phase 1 clinical trial of a Favored Health Organization birth control vaccine. Lancet 1988; 1295.

111. Wintsh J, Chaignut CL, Braun D, Jeannet M, Stalder H, Abrignani J, Montagna D, Chavijo F, Moret P, Dayer JM, Staehelin T, Doe B, Steimer KS, Dina D, Cruchaud A. Safety and immunogenicity of a genetically engineered human immunodeficiency virus vaccine. J Infect Dis 1991; 163:219.

VACCINE DEVELOPMENT: CURRENT STATUS/FUTURE DIRECTIONS

II

5

Contraceptive Vaccine Development

Future Prospects

Nancy J. Alexander*

Jones Institute for Reproductive Medicine
Eastern Virginia Medical School
Norfolk, Virginia

INTRODUCTION

Decisions on the utilization of the different fertility-regulating methods are dependent on the cultural, religious, socioeconomic, and health aspects of individuals. Availability of different methods varies from country to country, and thus decisions to use a certain contraceptive may be dictated

Current affiliation: National Institute of Child Health and Human Development, National Institutes of Health, Bethesda, Maryland.

This work was supported by the Contraceptive Research and Development Program (CONRAD), Eastern Virginia Medical School, under a Cooperative Agreement (DPE-2044-A-00-6063-00) with the United States Agency for International Development (A.I.D.). The views expressed by the author do not necessarily reflect the views of A.I.D.

not by individual preferences, but by methods that are prevalent in that country. While many highly efficacious methods of fertility regulation are currently available, additional methods of family planning in both developed and developing countries are needed.

Vaccines have been successfully utilized for over 150 years to control infectious diseases and have more recently been considered for other applications, including fertility regulation. Progress in contraceptive vaccine development has been stymied by many problems, including those associated with antigen identification, mass production, and efficacy and safety testing. Emergence of hybridoma and recombinant DNA technologies has been an important factor in facilitating the production of rare vaccine antigens, such as human proteins that can be employed in new vaccine approaches.

COMPARISON OF CONTRACEPTIVE AND TRADITIONAL VACCINES

There are many contrasts between contraceptive vaccines and more conventional vaccine approaches (1). Traditional vaccines provide protection against debilitating and often life-threatening diseases, whereas antifertility vaccines would be administered to healthy, fertile individuals to avoid unwanted pregnancy. Vaccines are often the only way to prevent an infectious disease, whereas for purposes of contraception there are a number of available methods. Traditional vaccines are to immunologically foreign antigens, whereas antifertility vaccines are directed against isologous antigens. These antigens associated with some aspect of reproduction may not be very immunogenic, and, in fact, some procedures may be required to break naturally acquired tolerance. Established vaccines are designed to generate a long-term, protective immunity, whereas vaccine-induced infertility should be for a shorter duration and should not produce permanent infertility. Therefore, natural exposure to the target antigen should not cause boosting.

A problem when developing a contraceptive vaccine is how to maintain effective antibody titers. With other vaccines, the immune system can rely on a memory response to the agent, but in the case of antifertility vaccines sufficient antibody must be present to quickly interrupt gamete interaction or affect hormone function. To maintain sufficiently high titers for prolonged infertility will probably require periodic administration of the antigen, by means of multiple injections or via some form of antigen-delivery system.

Termination of the contraceptive effect is another conundrum. In practice, it may be difficult to determine when the antibody titer has fallen to a level at which fertility is restored. The threshold fertility titer would be expected to show some variability, and person-to-person differences in the rate of titer decline would be expected. If a sperm antigen is utilized in a vaccine administered to women, a booster effect may develop after intercourse, prolonging the duration of infertility beyond the desired interval. Mechanisms to prevent or reverse this effect would have to be developed.

DEVELOPMENT OF A CONTRACEPTIVE VACCINE

The following steps in a fertility vaccine development have been suggested (1): 1) definition of the events or processes in reproduction accessible to immune intervention, 2) identification of molecules that when eliminated or neutralized will have an antifertility effect, 3) development of vaccines using natural or synthetic immunogens, 4) preclinical evaluations for efficacy and safety, and 5) clinical testing for safety and efficacy.

There are two major prerequisites for contraceptive vaccine use in human beings: 1) the antigen must be unique to the reproductive target and absent in other tissues, and 2) the antigen must have a fertility-related function.

Antigens associated with fertilization can be divided into at least three groups. These include the hypothalamic gonadotropin-releasing hormones (GnRH), pituitary gonadotropins [luteinizing hormone (LH) and follicle stimulating hormone (FSH)], gonadal steroids, and tissue-specific products of mature gametes and the early conceptus (Figure 1).

To date, research has focused on methods of immunizing women to prevent fertilization or early pregnancy. Since spermatozoa are foreign to the female tract, immunization with sperm-specific antigens appears to be a safer way to interfere with reproductive function than utilization of other antigens. In fact, some men and women do exhibit antisperm antibodies that can be linked to their infertility. Such findings, with no other untoward side effects, suggest that antibodies to sperm may affect fertility without a deleterious effect on other body functions. Laboratory studies have shown that immunization with a guinea pig sperm antigen results in 100% infertility in both male and female guinea pigs (2). However, definition of similar specific sperm antigens associated with human fertilization has lagged behind.

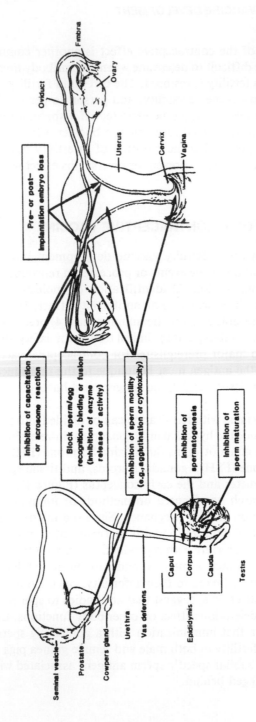

Figure 1 Some immunological antifertility effector mechanisms in the male and female reproductive systems. (From Simon LL, Alexander NJ. Sperm antigens as immunocontraceptives. In: Mathur S, Fredericks CM, eds. Perspectives in Immunoreproduction. New York: Hemisphere Publishing, 1988:224-241.)

Antigens in women that may have contraceptive potential include the vestments of the egg (Figure 2) that are produced late during oogenesis and are species-specific. Antibodies to the zona pellucida prevent spermatozoa from fertilizing the egg and appear to be the best target.

Neutralization of products produced by the developing conceptus has also been considered. In fact, the most extensive trials conducted to date are of an antifertility vaccine employing antigens based on the β subunit of human chorionic gonadotropin (hCG). This hormone, produced by syncytiotrophoblast cells, is essential in providing support to the corpus luteum during early gestation.

Which approach to contraception is best? The criteria for selecting candidate molecules include (1):

1. Relevance—immunological neutralizational results in infertility.
2. Specificity—cross-reactions with nontarget tissue that could lead to metabolic or immunopathological changes must not occur.

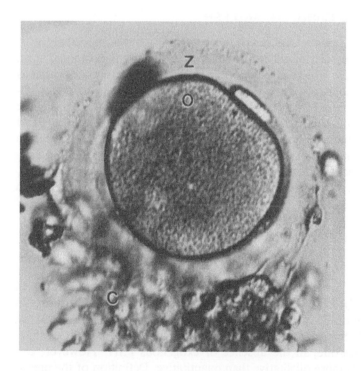

Figure 2   The human oocyte (O) is surrounded by a glycoprotein zona pelludica (Z) and cumulus cells (C). (Courtesy of L. Veeck.)

3. Accessibility—the target antigen must be accessible to antibodies and sensitized lymphocytes in the circulation or genital tract; the antigen must be secreted or expressed on the outer surface of the target cells.
4. Location—immune attack would best be concentrated in either the male or female tract such that systemic immune responses can be avoided.
5. Quantity—in order to avoid formation and deposition of insoluble immune complexes systemically, a small amount of antigen would be most appropriate.
6. Transience—ideally, antifertility vaccines should be directed against molecules that are only transiently present or found in low concentrations.
7. Synthesizability—the ability to prepare the immunogens by classic chemical synthesis or by recombinant DNA technology.

VACCINES TO GnRH, LH, AND FSH

Immunization against GnRH produces infertility but is associated with major endocrine disturbances. This approach has been considered for a vaccine for men. For libido to be maintained while spermatogenesis is suppressed, exogenous testosterone must be administered to males immunized with GnRH. With this regime, rats are unable to impregnate females although they exhibit normal sexual behavior (3). Both FSH and LH levels decline, and testis and epididymis weights decrease. The weights of the anterior pituitary, adrenals, and spleen remain normal. As antibody levels decline, hormone levels, organ weights, and fertility return. Since prostatic response to hormonal stimulation is reduced, this approach may be useful in the treatment of benign prostatic hyperplasia and prostatic tumors.

Normal testicular function is dependent on both LH and FSH. Whereas the role of LH as the essential hormone for the stimulation of steroidogenesis and, indirectly, spermatogenesis has been well defined, the role of FSH in the initiation and maintenance of spermatogenesis is less well understood (4). Initiation of spermatogenesis during puberty appears to be dependent on FSH, but its role during later stages of sexual life is less well defined. Spermatogenesis can be maintained by the male sex hormone, testosterone, in the absence of exogenous FSH. However, this maintenance is more qualitative than quantitative. Definition of the precise role of FSH has been hampered partially by the fact that FSH and LH preparations available for experimentation are not pure and each one contains some activity of the other.

Since FSH plays little role in testicular steroidogenesis, immunization against this hormone should not affect male sex function. Moudgal and co-workers (5,6) have conducted an extensive number of immunization experiments in laboratory animals, including nonhuman primates, that indicate that reversible infertility can be produced in the male. A vaccine consisting of ovine FSH and alum has produced consistent infertility in both bonnet (6) and cynomolgus monkeys (7) without any apparent effect on mating behavior. A spontaneous return to fertility after a 2-3-year period of infertility has been observed (6,8). This return to fertility is observed even with continuing high anti-FSH antibody titers. The precise reason for this occurrence is not understood. Perhaps small amounts of FSH elute from the alum hydrogel backbone and stimulate spermatogenesis, but why this does not occur following earlier boostings with the vaccine is not clear. Whether this unacceptable problem can be circumvented through the use of a vaccine based on only the β-subunit of FSH is not known, although the use of the subunit is an attractive idea.

Toxicological evaluation of the ovine FSH vaccine in rodents and nonhuman primates has failed to reveal any pathological findings in the numerous tissues that were examined. As a heterologous antigen, ovine FSH may be more antigenic in primates than native FSH. However, it remains to be established whether FSH derived from pituitary glands of sheep is acceptable from the standpoint of safety for human experimentation. Nevertheless, based on animal experiments, the anti-FSH vaccine represents a potential approach to the regulation of male fertility.

Vaccination against LH has not been given serious consideration as a means of regulating fertility in either the male or the female. In addition to the inhibition of both gametogenesis and steroidogenesis, similar to what is observed with the anti-GnRH vaccine, the approach involves the utilization of a protein molecule that is much more complex than a simple decapeptide like GnRH. From a strictly practical standpoint, production of GnRH for vaccine utilization is a much simpler process than the isolation of LH from pituitaries or its generation through recombinant DNA technology.

VACCINES TO hCG

The most extensively studied vaccines are based on antibodies to hCG. Since pituitary gonadotropins and hCG have a similar α-subunit, antibodies to the whole hCG molecule cross-react with both LH and FSH, thus making a vaccine based on the whole hCG molecule of limited utility. The β-subunit differs among the various gonadotropins, and a vaccine based on this subunit offers greater specificity. However, some cross-reactivity with LH has been observed in clinical studies (9).

The C-terminal region of β-hCG is unique to this subunit, and antibodies to it do not cross-react with LH. However, the C-terminus peptide is less immunogenic and must be conjugated to a larger carrier molecule in order to elicit effective antibody titers. A series of peptides have been synthesized representing sequences from six to 47 amino acids of the C-terminus. Peptides of fewer than 20 amino acids were generally less immunogenic. Furthermore, the use of small peptides as immunogens resulted in antibodies incapable of neutralizing the biological activity of hCG (10). Peptides more than 35 residues in length consistently produced antibodies capable of neutralizing hCG; therefore, only peptides of this length or longer were considered for vaccine development by the WHO scientists. Various carriers have been tested, including bovine gamma-globulin, tetanus toxoid, and diptheria toxoid; since diphtheria toxoids elicited fewer delayed-type hypersensitivity reactions, it was chosen for further vaccine development. Adjuvants and delivery systems have also been considered. Muramyl dipeptide analogs were compared to complete Freund's adjuvant, as were a variety of oil-and-water emulsions (11).

Adult female baboons have been immunized with a number of different peptide conjugates and adjuvants. Females mated with males of proven fertility had a significant reduction in their fertility rate (12,13). Following the baboon antifertility trials, toxicity testing in rodents and immunosafety tests in baboons were conducted. Immune complexes, hormone levels, antibody binding to normal tissues, and histopathological examination of tissues from immunized animals were evaluated. In a phase I clinical trial conducted in Australia, young, healthy women who had previously been sterilized by tubal ligation received various doses of the vaccine. The vaccine strategy adopted by the WHO Task Force on Fertility Regulating Vaccines involved the use of the synthetic peptide corresponding to the amino acid sequence 109 to 145 of the β-hCG molecule. The components of the vaccine included a water-soluble synthetic MDP analog as an adjuvant and a saline oil emulsion vehicle that consisted of four parts squalene to one part mannide mono-oleate (ARLA-A) as an emulsifying agent. Thirty-three women who had been surgically sterilized were assigned to five dosage groups of six each and received the vaccine by intramuscular injection on two occasions, 6 weeks apart. It became apparent that without the use of a carrier, frequent immunization would be necessary to maintain contraceptive levels (14). The study revealed that significant levels of antibodies to hCG were attained. Animal teratology studies are under way, and a Phase II clinical efficacy study is being planned.

While the WHO approach to an anti-hCG vaccine has been based exclusively on the C-terminal peptide, the Population Council and the Indian National Institute of Immunology (NII) have focused on a variety of vaccines based on the whole β-subunit. The latter two organizations opted for the greater antigenicity of the whole subunit, with a slight sacrifice in specificity. Extensive Phase I clinical studies have been conducted by NII in order to select the best candidate for efficacy trials. It now appears that a vaccine based on β-hCG linked to tetanus toxoid may be a viable candidate for future studies. A potential problem of utilizing tetanus toxoid as a carrier arose when some women developed hypersensitivity to the carrier as the result of previous immunizations with this toxoid. This may necessitate switching to diphtheria toxoid as an alternative carrier (15).

The maintenance of effective anti-hCG antibody levels requires periodic boosting. While this approach may be viable in controlled clinical studies, it represents a stumbling point if the vaccine approach is to be utilized for mass immunization programs. Consequently, research on the development of vaccine delivery systems that could obviate periodic boosting and result in prolonged high levels of antibodies has been initiated. Experiments have been designed to ascertain whether sustained antibody levels can best be obtained by bursts of antigen delivery or continuous release, and whether adjuvant is necessary during the period of antibody production. Antigen availability results in high antibody levels, and consistent release is immunogenic and not tolerogenic. Therefore, it is not necessary for adjuvant to be continuously present; it is probably not essential after the first few days of the primary immunization (16). Oil emulsion systems, liposomes, and ISCOMS were evaluated, but by far the best approach was the development of a biodegradable microsphere system. The idea is that it will be necessary to have sustained antibody levels for a period of at least one year. Without the use of biodegradable microsystems, several injections were required to sustain effective levels of antibodies even for several months (16).

ZONA PELLUCIDA ANTIGENS

Oogenesis occurs during fetal life, but final maturation is completed shortly before ovulation. During this maturation period, production of specialized antigenic substances could provide possible targets for immunocontraception. Unlike the zona pellucida (ZP), the cumulus and corona cells do not express tissue-specific antigens (Figure 2). All cell types in the ovary are exposed to the full range of serum components, including antibodies, so an antigen-antibody response can occur. In fact, antibodies to ovarian antigens, including those of the ZP, may be responsible for certain naturally occurring infertility problems (17,18). Antibodies to the zona can inhibit both attachment of sperm to the ZP surface and sperm penetration (19,20).

Initially, the noncellular glycoprotein ZP appears as small patches in the vicinity of the microvilli of the oocyte membrane and adjacent granulosa cell membranes and is deposited in patches that coalesce to form a continuous layer (21). The developing oocyte is capable of synthesizing all the components of the ZP (22-24), but cultures of granulosa cells also demonstrate the ability to secrete ZP material (25). This layer surrounding the mature oocyte is probably jointly synthesized and secreted by follicular cells as well as the growing oocyte.

Zona pellucida binding with sperm is the first step in sperm-egg interaction. Studies have shown that exposure of zona to polyclonal antizona antisera prevents sperm attachment. Extensive studies of mouse ZP proteins indicate the presence of three glycoprotein families—ZP1, ZP2, and ZP3—composed of asparagine-linked complex-type oligosaccarides; at least two of these also contain serine/threonine-linked carbohydrates (26). A specific class of 0-linked oligosaccharides on the ZP3 molecule containing an α-linked galactose at the nonreducing terminus functions as the initial attachment site for sperm through galactosyl transferase activity residing on the sperm surface (27). These carbohydrate side chains of the zona proteins are very important in determining immunogenicity and contraceptive efficacy. Immunization with the complete ZP3 results in high titers of antizona antibodies, whereas immunization with the purified core proteins generates a reduced or undetectable antibody response (28). Therefore, the biochemical composition of the carbohydrate side chains must be elucidated to determine the mechanisms by which these structures define antigenicity.

The immune response generated against ZP proteins often produces effects on the ovary unrelated to the inhibition of the sperm-ZP interaction, namely, autoimmune oophoritis. The large antral follicles producing steroids do not develop probably because the ZP matrix does not establish normal contact with the cells of the developing follicle. Total depletion of germ cells and follicles may occur (29). Vaccines must be engineered to disturb ovarian function and steroidogenesis minimally and yet provide reversible suppression of fertility. Two recent studies indicate that this is possible. No ovarian damage was observed in horses immunized with solubilized porcine ZP, and 14 of 16 mares were infertile (31). In another study, mice immunized with a 16-amino-acid peptide of ZP3 developed antizona antibodies and reversible infertility without ovarian damage (31). Understanding and separating the B-cell response directed to zona proteins and the T-cell response that may result in cytotoxicity is important. Vaccine strategies based on immunization with ZP peptides containing only B-cell epitopes are being devised (31).

SPERM ANTIGENS

Spermatozoa are unique haploid cells that express gene products not found in cells elsewhere on the body. Although these molecules are potent autoantigens, they rarely induce immune responses because sperm and germ cells are separated, at least to some extent, from the immune system by the blood-testis barrier.

Epididymal Antigens

Mammalian spermatozoa continue to develop as they pass through the epididymis. New antigens coat the spermatozoa during epididymal transit. Immature spermatozoa from the proximal epididymal segments gain the ability to bind to the ZP and fertilize ova after being incubated with preparations of secreted epididymal glycoproteins (32-34). Human sperm also develop the capacity to penetrate zona-free hamster eggs as they pass through successive segments of the human epididymis (35). Such data suggest that epididymal antigens are fertility-regulating factors and that antibodies to such molecules could result in infertility. Antisera to epididymal antigens have been produced and when exposed to human sperm provide in vitro evidence of fertility reduction (36). Motility parameters are not altered by the antisera, and agglutination affects only 7% of the motile cells; therefore, inhibition of hamster ova penetration is not due to these changes. Indeed, such studies suggest that the antisera bind to the sperm surface and interfere with attachment of the spermatozoa to the oolema (37).

Epididymal proteins associated with maturing spermatozoa may possess the requisite specificity for a true block to male fertility. One protein purified from the rat epididymis and utilized for immunization has a molecular weight of 37,000, is androgen-dependent, and is produced by the epithelium of the proximal segments of the epididymis (37). Ultrastructural studies reveal that this antigen is localized on the external surface of the sperm plasma membrane, covering the acrosomal and post-acrosomal regions of the head (38). Antibodies to this protein affect hamster egg penetration, suggesting that the antigen plays a specific role in

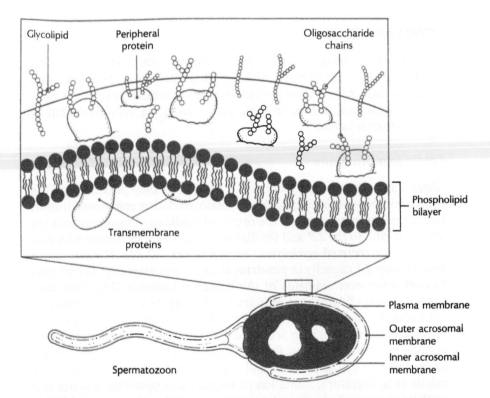

Figure 3   The plasma membrane of the spermatozoon overlays an acrosome composed of the outer acrosomal and inner acrosomal membranes. After the acrosome reaction, lysis and fusion of these membranes allow exposure of new membrane antigens of the inner acrosomal membranes. (From Alexander NJ. Natural and induced immunological infertility. Curr Opinion Immunol 1989; 1: 1120-1130.)

the interaction of the sperm with oolema. Since coating antigens are on the sperm surface, the use of antibodies to such agents could be an important approach to contraception.

Antigens of Ejaculated Spermatozoa

Specific domains (Figure 3) are created from the time the sperm are formed in the testis, and these may change and shift during passage through the male reproductive tract and finally in the female reproductive fluids. Sperm, upon ejaculation, continue to undergo a series of maturational steps. These steps involve changes in membrane fluidity, most likely due to the depletion of membrane cholesterol. This decrease in the cholesterol-to-phospholipid molar ratio (39) leads to changes in such membrane properties as ionic permeability. The mammalian sperm surface is heterogeneous (Figure 4). A variety of probes have been used to detect an uneven

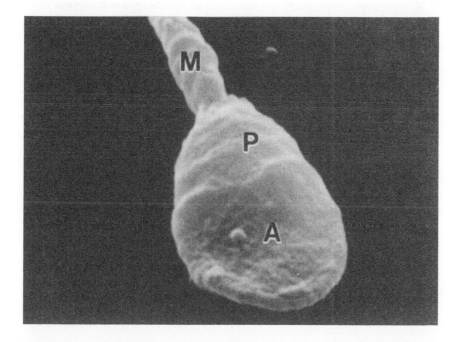

Figure 4 A scanning electron micrograph of human spermatozoon. (A) Acrosome; (P) postacrosomal region; (M) midpiece composed of helical array of mitochondria. Sperm antigens are often localized to distinct regions. 15,000×.

distribution of surface charges, including lectin binding groups (Figure 5), antibody binding sites (Figures 6a and 6b), and intramembrane particles as revealed by freeze-fracture (40). Membrane molecules can be either an integral or a peripheral part of the membrane. Maintenance of sperm-surface domains depends on this distribution. Restriction of molecular diffusion may occur because molecules are tethered in a particular position or because a barrier in the membrane does not allow free diffusion of molecules from one surface to another (40).

Another confounding factor in the study of sperm antigens is their heterogeneity; spermatozoa in an ejaculate may be at several maturational stages. This heterogeneity ensures that some spermatozoa may be at an appropriate stage at the time of sperm and egg interaction, which in turn ensures that fertilization will occur, enhancing preservation of

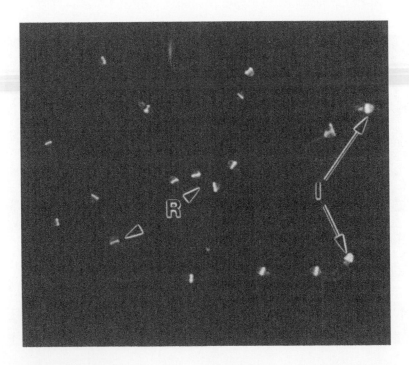

Figure 5 Human spermatozoa stained with the lectin FITC-PNS. Acrosome-reacted sperm appear as a bar (R), and acrosome intact (I) exhibit fluorescence over the acrosome. 800×.

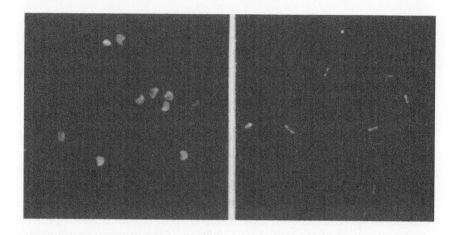

Figure 6 Serum samples that react solely with (left) the acrosome of human sperm and (right) the equatorial region of human sperm. 900×.

the species. For the scientist, this heterogeneity makes studies of sperm antigen localization more difficult.

As domains are shifted, some molecules are eliminated from the surface and some moved from one region to another. The acrosome reaction results in a major rearrangement of the plasma membrane. Molecules in the interior head are shed from the cell, and a new membrane, potentially with a different set of molecules, becomes the surface. Studies over the years reveal the necessity of the acrosome reaction for fertilization in all species examined. Even when presented with an egg denuded of its coverings, the plasma membranes of sperm that have not acrosome-reacted are unable to fuse. Sperm that undergo a premature acrosome reaction are excluded from further participation in fertilization. Those that acrosome-react before reaching the cumulus are unable to enter the matrix (42,43).

Coating antigens of seminal plasma, in addition to those of the epididymis, are involved with fertilization. In fact, sperm-immobilizing antibodies in the sera of some infertile women have been found to react with components of human seminal plasma (44). A monoclonal antibody has been generated by fusing lymphocytes from a woman with antisperm antibodies. The use of this monoclonal antibody has allowed definition of a carbohydrate antigen that presumably is responsible for the infertility (45).

Only a few sperm-specific antigens (i.e., protamine, lactate dehydrogenase-C4 (LDH-C4), RS-1, acrosin) have been extensively characterized. Several laboratories have recently developed monoclonal antibodies to a variety of sperm antigens and are using them to identify and characterize new sperm proteins.

LDH-C4

The best defined sperm antigen is LDH-C4, an isoenzyme of lactate dehydrogenase found only in male germ cells. This glycolytic enzyme exists in multiple molecular forms, or isozymes, that consist of subunit types A, B, and C. These subunits, each with a distinctive gene product, combine as homo- or heterotetrameric proteins with distinct tissue and functional specificities (46). LDH-C4 first appears with onset of puberty during prophase of the first meotic division of the primary spermatocyte (47) and is found on mature spermatozoa. LDH-C4 is never synthesized by females and is sequestered from the immune system of the male by the blood-testis barrier. Immunization of both males and females with purified LDH-C4 provokes an immune response. Antibodies to LDH-C4 partially suppress fertility in female mice, rabbits, and baboons (49,50). The antibodies cause some agglutination and, in some cases, complement mediated cell lysis. Since oviductal fluids are a transudate of serum, high circulating-antibody levels probably result in sufficient quantities of antibody in the oviducts. Ovulatory cycles are not affected by immunization, nor are there any other deleterious side effects. Sperm antigens such as LDH-C4 cannot be used as vaccines in males because orchitis often develops.

The antigen was first isolated in gram amounts from mouse testis (51). When the amino acid sequence of the subunit became known (52), it was then possible to map antigenic determinants of the molecule by synthesizing a panel of peptides chosen according to criteria of surface accessibility, flexibility, and evolutionary variability (53). One of the synthetic vaccines, conjugated to diphtheria toxoid, induced a specific immune response to the native protein as well as a protective immunity against pregnancies. Only three pregnancies occurred among 14 female baboons immunized with this synthetic peptide (54). Next, a cDNA expression library packaged in lambda gt11 was screened with polyclonal and monoclonal antibodies to murine LDH-C4 (55). This allowed deduction of the amino acid sequence for human LDH-C4, which had a sequence similarity of 74% to that for mouse LDH-C4. The cDNA was engineered for expression in *E. coli*. The Goldberg group has successfully engineered the human ldh cDNA to produce a recombinant vaccinia that expresses LDH-C4 (56). The next obvious step is a fertility trial in baboons. Such a trial is currently being initiated.

Protamine

Protamine, which replaces histones in the sperm nucleus during spermiogenesis, is a sperm-specific autoantigen that elicits antibodies in 30% of vasectomized men, but it is not a likely candidate for a sperm vaccine since it is internally located. LDH-C4 is also an internal antigen, but it appears to leak through the plasma membrane and thus is accessible, to some extent, to antibodies.

Acrosin

The serine protease acrosin is located in the mammalian sperm acrosome. Present as proacrosin from the early spermatid stage (57), this enzyme is also involved in the acrosome reaction and dispersion of the acrosomal matrix (57) and is important in binding and penetration of the spermatozoa across the zona pellucida. Since acrosin is exposed after the acrosome reaction, it appears to be functional after initial gamete binding (58). Gamete binding to mouse zonae can be dissected into two steps (59,60). The first involves interaction of the receptor located on the plasma membrane, with ZP3 probably inducing the acrosome reaction. Complementary receptor molecules present on both gametes allow for fusion at the sperm-zona interface (61). After binding to the zona, sperm undergo the acrosome reaction allowing for the release of proteolytic enzymes that enable the sperm to traverse the zona. The second step involves a receptor located on the inner acrosomal membrane exposed only after the acrosome reaction. With the acrosome reaction, ZP3 is released together with the plasma membrane, and the sperm remain bound to the zona through the ZP2 receptor. Acrosin appears to participate in the controlled digestion of the ZP3 and ZP2. Sperm acrosin appears in an inactive zymogen form of proacrosin with a molecular weight of 53,000-55,000 (62,63). Proacrosin is activated by an intrazymogen mechanism rather than by the influence of an activating protease (64). Proacrosin can interact with carbohydrate moeities of the zona glycoproteins, and thus it may play a role in the secondary binding of reacted sperm through a fucose binding site (65).

Fucoidin strongly inhibits sperm-zona binding (66-68), and fucose, in a confirmation similar to that of fucoidin, has been suggested to be part of the recognition between gametes (69). After induction of the acrosome reaction by the calcium ionophore A23187, there is a dramatic exposure or activation of fucose binding sites (70). Fucose binding activity may be associated with components of the acrosome. Some investigators think that the spatial α-1-3 linkage of the monosaccharides, fucose, galactose, or glucose, and the position of the sulfate on the C4 carbon along the backbone of the molecule, are more important than the specific monosaccharide (71).

RSA-1

RSA-1 is a sperm-specific antigen found on pachytene spermatocytes and on the plasma membrane of rabbit sperm. RSA peptides obtained from a 14,000 kDa family are autoantigenic and may be involved with sperm binding (71). Some individuals with immunologically mediated infertility have antibodies to RSA-1 (72).

SP-10

In 1986, the World Health Organization Task Force on Contraceptive Vaccines held a workshop to define monoclonal antibodies that seemed to recognize sperm-specific antigens that could be considered vaccine candidates. Several major monoclonal candidates were defined, and one of them was identified as MHS-10. The antigen to MHS-10, SP-10, is located on human testicular germ cells and is an abundant surface antigen on mature sperm. The monoclonal exhibits minimal or no cross-reactivity with somatic cells. The antigen is first detected in round spermatids as ovoid granules and later becomes associated with the nascent acrosomal granule. However, SP-10 is not on the outer plasma membrane of intact sperm but in the inner acrosomal membrane (73). Some could think that the location in an intraacrosomal membrane would diminish the potential of SP-10 as a vaccine immunogen, but SP-10 remains associated with the sperm head following the acrosome reaction. If antibodies are present in sufficient numbers, further penetration of the zona could be impeded.

After the acrosome reaction, the acrosomal contents are externalized and the inner acrosomal membrane becomes the limiting membrane of the anterior sperm head. The number of acrosome-reacted sperm on the zona increases rapidly (74). After penetration of the zona, fusion of the sperm and egg occurs between the plasma membrane over the equatorial segment of the spermatozoon and the egg plasma membrane. If antibodies in the secretions of the female tract can gain access to antigens on the inner acrosomal membrane, blockage of sperm-egg fusion would be expected. Molecular characterization of SP-10 by Western blots reveals resolution of at least 14 distinctive immunoreactive sperm peptide bands ranging in molecular weight from 18,000 to 34,000. SP-10 can be found in the sperm of other primates, an important consideration when considering animal-testing possibilities for vaccine efficacy and safety.

HS-11 and HS-63

These monoclonals react specifically with the sperm acrosome of mammalian species and do not react with other somatic tissues. The mouse antigen equivalent is immunogenic in mice and rabbits and causes an anti-fertility effect. Molecular cloning of the sperm antigen gene has been accomplished and a recombinant fusion protein has been obtained (75).

A Polyclonal Sperm-Specific Antigen

Another approach to define sperm antigens has been the use of poly-clonal antibodies (71,76-79). One polyclonal of particular interest reacts with the acrosome. This evolutionarily conserved acrosomal antigen causes strong sperm agglutination and fertility reduction in mice and monkeys (76). The antigen is of approximately 40 kD in human sperm and 69 kD in monkey sperm. Antibodies raised against the blot antigens reveal similar immune responses to the original polyclonal antibody. Immunization with the antigen impedes fertility.

CONCLUSION

This chapter attempts to define the current status of research on contraceptive vaccines. Fertility regulation represents a unique aspect of therapeutics. It is an attempt to regulate a very normal and indispensable function of the human race, namely, reproduction. With the advent of oral contraceptives, the concept of chemical control of fertility has become well established. The early history of oral contraceptives is well documented and is replete with allegations concerning serious hazards of this approach. While numerous side effects of oral contraceptives, from serious ones such as cancer to many more benign ones, are still the subject of scientific studies, the overall safety and benefits far outweigh the real and presumed risks.

Development of contraceptive vaccines is still in its infancy. Identification of specific antigens and their full chemical and immunological characterization is a difficult scientific endeavor. Demonstration that antigens isolated from tissues of laboratory animals have their counterparts in human cells is mandatory. Clinical experimentation is limited to the vaccines based on β-hCG or its fragments. Efficacy testing must be combined with adequate experimentation to determine the potential safety of a product.

The research and development process for antifertility vaccines is complex. Consequently, it must be appreciated that this approach to fertility regulation will require considerable investment in time and resources before its complete potential can be realized. However, the scientific and programatic difficulties are not insurmountable, and the potential benefits that antifertility vaccines offer are substantial. Additionally, the area of antifertility vaccine development represents a unique situation in terms of international collaboration. Scientists from developing nations in collaboration with their counterparts from developed countries have played a major role in advancing this scientific frontier.

ACKNOWLEDGMENTS

My thanks to Gabriel Bialy, Ph.D., for his constructive suggestions in the preparation of this manuscript and my appreciation to Diane P. Spencer for typing this manuscript.

REFERENCES

1. Griffin D. Strategy of vaccine development. In: Alexander NJ, Griffin PD, Spieler M, Waites GMH, eds. Gamete Interaction: Prospects for Immunocontraception. New York: Wiley-Liss, 1990:503-524.
2. Primakoff P, Lathrop W, Woodman L, Cowan A, Myles D. Fully effective contraception in female guinea pigs immunized with the sperm protein PH-20. Nature 1988; 335:543-546.
3. Ladd A, Tsong Y-Y, Prabhu G, Thau A. Effects of long-term immunization against LHRH and androgen treatment on gonadal function. J Reprod Immunol 1989; 15:85-101.
4. Bremner WJ, Matsumotoa AM. Endocrine control of human spermatogenesis: possible mechanism for contraception. In: Zatuchni GI, Goldsmith A, Spieler JM, Sciarra JJ, eds. Male Contraception Advances and Future Prospects. Philadelphia: Harper & Row, 1986:81-88.
5. Moudgal NR. A need for FSH in maintaining fertility of adult male subhuman primates. Arch Androl 1981; 7:117-125.
6. Moudgal NR, Murthy GS, Rao AL, et al. Development of oFSH as a vaccine for the male—a status report on the recent researches carried out using the bonnet monkey *M. radiata*. In: Talwar GP, ed. Proceedings of the International Symposium on Immunological Approaches to Contraception and Promotion of Fertility. New York: Plenum Press, 1986:103-110.

7. Madhwa Raj HG. Effects of active immunization with follicle stimulating hormone (FSH) on spermatogenesis in the adult-crab eating monkey—evaluation for male contraception. In: Talwar GP, ed. Immunological Approaches to Contraception and Promotion of Fertility. New York: Plenum Press, 1986:115-123.

8. Nieschlag E. Reasons for abandoning immunization against FSH as an approach to male fertility regulation. In: Zatuchni GI, Goldsmith A, Spieler JM, Sciarra JJ, eds. Male Contraception: Advances and Future Prospects. Philadelphia: Harper & Row, 1986:395-400.

9. Kharat E, Nair NS, Dhall K, et al. Analysis of menstrual records of women immunized with anti-hCG vaccines inducing antibodies partially cross-reactive with hLH. Contraception 1990; 41:293-299.

10. Stevens VC. Development of hCG antifertility vaccine. In: Mathur S, Fredericks CM, eds. Perspectives in Immunoreproduction. New York: Hemisphere Publishing, 1988:205-223.

11. Stevens VC, Cinader B, Powell JE, Lee AC, Koh SW. Preparation and formulation of a hCG antifertility vaccine: Selection of an adjuvant and vehicle. Am J Reprod Immunol 1981; 6:315-321.

12. Stevens VC. Human choronic gonadotropin: properties and potential immunological manipulation for clinical application. In: Jones W, ed. Clinics of Obstetrics and Gynecology. Vol. 6. London: WB Saunders 1979:549-566.

13. Talwar GP, Gupta SK, Tandon AK. Immunologic interruption of pregnancy. In: Gleicher N, ed. Reproductive Immunology. New York: Alan R Liss, 1981: 451-460.

14. Jones WR. Lessons from an anti-hCG contraceptive vaccine trial. In: Alexander NJ, Griffin PD, Spieler JM, Waites GMH, eds. Gamete Interaction: Prospects for Immunocontraception. New York: Wiley-Liss, 1990:597-608.

15. Talwar GP, Singh O, Pal R, Arunan K. Experiences of the anti-hCG vaccine of relevance to development of other birth control vaccines. In: Alexander NJ, Griffin PD, Spieler JM, Waites GMH, eds. Gamete Interaction: Prospects for Immunocontraception. New York: Wiley-Liss, 1990:581-596.

16. Stevens VC, Powell JE, Rickey M, Lee AC, Lewis DH. Studies of various delivery systems for a hCG vaccine. In: Alexander NJ, Griffin PD, Spieler JM, Waites GMH, eds. Gamete Interaction: Prospects for Immunocontraception. New York: Wiley-Liss, 1990:551-566.

17. Damewood MD, Zacur HA, Hoffman GJ, Rock JA. Circulating antiovarian antibodies in premature ovarian failure. Obstet Gynecol 1986; 68:850-854.

18. Mignot MH, Schoemaker J, Kleingeld M, Roa BR, Drexhage HA. Premature ovarian failure. I. The association with autoimmunity. Eur J Gynecol Reprod Biol 1989; 30:59-66.

19. Dunbar BS, Wolgemuth DJ. Structure and function of the mammalian zona pellucida, a unique extracellular matrix. In: Satir B, ed. Modern Cell Biology. New York: Alan R.Liss, 1984:77-111.

20. Henderson CJ, Braude P, Aitken RJ. Polyclonal antibodies to a 32-KDa deglycosylated polypeptide from porcine zonae pellucidae will prevent human gamete interaction in vitro. Gamete Res 1987; 18:251-265.

21. Sacco AG. Development and maturation of the zona pellucida. In: Alexander NJ, Griffin PD, Spieler JM, Waites GMH, eds. Gamete Interaction: Prospects for Immunocontraception. New York: Wiley-Liss, 1990:261-278.

22. Bleil JD, Wassarman PM. Structure and function of the zona pellucida: Identification and characterization of the proteins of the mouse oocyte's zona pellucida. Develop Biol 1980; 76:185-202.

23. Greve JM, Salzmann GS, Roller RJ. Wassarman PM. Biosynthesis of the major zona pellucida glycoprotein secreted by oocytes during mammalian oogenesis. Cell 1982; 31:749-759.

24. Shimizu S, Tsuji M, Dean J. In vitro biosynthesis of three sulfated glycoproteins of murine zonae pellucidae by oocytes grown in follicle culture. J Biol Chem 1983; 258:5858-5863.

25. Maresh GA, Dunbar BS. Expression of specific proteins by ovarian primary follicles cultured in vitro. Biol Reprod 1987(suppl 1); 36:88a.

26. Wassarman PM. Zona pellucida glycoproteins. Ann Rev Biochem 1988; 57: 415-442.

27. Macek MB, Shur BD. Protein-carbohydrate complementarity in mammalian gamete recognition. Gamete Res 1988; 20:93-109.

28. Aitken RJ, Paterson M, Braude P, Thillai Koothan P. Evaluation of glycosylated and deglycosylated porcine zona antigens for contraceptive efficacy in vivo and in vitro. In: Alexander NJ, Griffin PD, Spieler JM, Waites GMH, eds. Gamete Interaction: Prospects for Immunocontraception. New York: Wiley-Liss, 1990:295-314.

29. Timmons TM, Skinner SM, Dunbar BS. Glycosylation and maturation of the mammalian zona pellucida. In: Alexander NJ, Griffin PD, Spieler JM, Waites GMH, eds. Gamete Interaction: Prospects of Immunocontraception. New York: Wiley-Liss, 1990:279-294.

30. Liu IKM, Bernoco M, Feldman M. Contraception in mares heteroimmunized with pig zonae pellucidae. J Reprod Fertil 1989; 85:19-29.

31. Millar SE, Chamow SM, Balir AW, Oliver C, Robey F, Dean J. Vaccination with a synthetic zona pellucida peptide produces long-term contraception in female mice. Science 1989; 246:935-938.

32. Cuasnicu P, Gonzalez Echeverria F, Piazza A, Cameo M, Blaquier J. Antibodies against epididymal glycoproteins block fertilizing ability in rat. J Reprod Fert 1984; 72:467-471.

33. Moore H, Hartman T. In vitro development of the fertilizing ability of hamster epididymal spermatozoa after co-culture with epithelium from the proximal cauda epididymis. J Reprod Fert 1986; 78:347-353.

34. Orgebin-Crist MC, Fournier-Delpech S. Sperm-egg interaction. Evidence for maturational changes during epididymal transit. J Androl 1982; 3:429-433.

35. Hinrichsen MJ, Blaquier JA. Evidence supporting the existence of sperm maturation in the human epididymis. J Reprod Fert 1980; 60:291-294.

36. Cameo MS, Dawidowski A, Sanjuruo C, Gonzalez Escheverria F, Blaquier JA. Changes in sperm specific antigens during epididymal maturation. In: Alexander NJ, Griffin PD, Spieler JM, Waites GMH, eds. Gamete Interaction: Prospects for Immunocontraception. New York: Wiley-Liss, 1990: 129-142.

37. Gaberi JC, Kohane AC, Cameo MS, Blaquier JA. Isolation and characterization of specific rat epididymal proteins. Molec Cell Endor 1979; 13:73-82.

38. Cameo MS, Gonzalez Echeverria F, Blaquier JA, Burgos M. Immunochemical localization of epididymal protein DE on rat spermatozoa: Its fate after induced acrosome reaction. Gamete Res 1986; 15:247-257.

39. Davis BK. Timing of fertilization in mammals: sperm cholesterol/phospholipid ratio as a determinant of the capacitation interval. Proc Natl Acad Sci USA 1981; 78:7560-7564.

40. Myles DG, Koppel DE, Primakoff P. Defining sperm surface domains. In: Alexander NJ, Griffin PD, Spieler JM, Waites GMH, eds. Gamete Interaction: Prospects for Immunocontraception. New York: Wiley-Liss, 1990:1-12.

41. Yanagimachi R. Mammalian fertilization. In: Knobil E, Neill J, eds. Physiology of Reproduction. Vol 1. New York: Raven Press, 1987:135-185.

42. Cherr G, Lambert H, Meizel W, Katz D. In vitro studies of the golden hamster sperm acrosome reaction: completion on the zona pellucida and induction by homologous soluble zonae pellucidae. Devel Biol 1986; 114:119-131.

43. Cummins J, Yanagimachi R. Development of ability to penetrate the cumulus oophorus by hamster spermatozoa capacitated in vitro, in relation to the timing of the acrosome reaction. Gamete Res 1986; 15:187-212.

44. Isojima S, Li TS, Ashitaka Y. Immunologic analysis of sperm-immobilizing factor found in sera of women with unexplained sterility. Am J Obst Gynec 1968; 101:677-683.

45. Isojima S, Kameda K, Koyama K, Batova I, Tsuji Y. Development of heterohybridomas to define human sperm coating antigen. In: Alexander NJ, Griffin PD, Spieler JM, Waites GMH, eds. Gamete Interaction: Prospects for Immunocontraception. New York: Wiley-Liss, 1990:361-378.

46. Markert CL. Isozomes in kidney development. In: Metcoff J, ed. Hereditary Development and Immunologic Aspects of Kidney Disease. Chicago: Northwestern University Press, 1962:54-64.

47. Hintz M, Goldberg E. Immunohistochemical localization of LDH-X during spermatogenesis in mouse testes. Devel Biol 1977; 57:375-384.

48. Goldberg E. Isozymes in testes and spermatozoa. In: Rattazzi MC, Scandalios JG, Whitt GS, eds. Isozymes: Current Topics in Biological and Medical Research. Vol. 1. New York: Alan R Liss, 1977:79-124.

49. Goldberg E. Lactate dehydrogenase-X (crystalline) from mouse testes. In: Methods in Enzymology. Vol. XLI. Carbohydrate Metabolism. Part B. New York: Academic Press, 1975:318-322.

50. Wheat TE, Goldberg E. Sperm-specific lactate dehydrogenase C₄: Antigenic structure and immuno-suppression of fertility. In: Retezzi MC, Scandalios JG, Whitt GS, eds. Isozymes: Current Topics in Biological and Medical Research. Vol. 7. New York: Alan R Liss, 1983:113-130.

51. Lee CY, Huan JH, Goldberg E. Lactate dehydrogenase from the mouse. In: Wood WA, ed. Carbohydrate Metabolism. Part D. Methods in Enzymology. New York: Academic Press, 1982:351-362.

52. Hogrefe HH, Griffith JP, Rossmann MG, Goldberg E. Characterization of antigenic sites on the refined 3A structure of mouse testicular lactate dehydrogenase-C4. J Biol Chem 1987; 262:13155-13162.

53. Hogrefe HH, Kaumaya PTP, Goldberg E. Immunogenicity of synthetic peptides corresponding to flexible and antibody-accessible segments of mouse lactate dehydrogenase (LDH)-C₄. J Biol Chem 1989; 264:10513-10519.

54. Wheat TE, Goldberg E. Antigenic domains of the sperm-specific lactate dehydrogenase C₄ isozyme. Mol Immunol 1985; 22:643-649.

55. Millan JL, Driscoll CE, LeVan KM, Goldberg E. Epitopes of human testis-specific lactate dehydrogenase deduced from a cDNA sequence. Proc Natl Acad Sci USA 1987; 84:5311-5315.

56. Goldberg E. LDH-C4 as an immunocontraceptive model. In: Alexander NJ, Griffin PD, Spieler JM, Waites GMH, eds. Gamete Interaction: Prospects for Immunocontraception. New York: Wiley-Liss, 1990:63-74.

57. Dunbar BS, Dudkiewicz AB, Bundman DS. Proteolysis of specific procine zona pellucida glycoproteins by boar acrosin. Biol Reprod 1985; 32:619-630.

58. Saling PM. Mammalian sperm interaction with extracellular matrices of the egg. Oxford Rev Reprod Biol 1989; 11:339-388.

59. Bleil J, Wassarman PM. Autoradiographic visualization of the mouse egg sperm receptor bound to sperm. J Cell Biol 1986; 102:1363-1371.

60. Bleil JD, Greve JM, Wassarman PM. Identification of a secondary sperm receptor in the mouse egg zona pellucida: role in maintenance of binding of acrosome-reacted sperm to egg. Dev Biol 1988; 128:376-385.

61. O'Rand MG. Sperm-egg recognition and barriers to interspecies fertilization. Gamete Res 1988; 19:315-328.

62. Cechova D, Topfer-Petersen E, Henschen A. Boar acrosin is a single-chain molecule which has the N-terminus of the acrosin A-chain (light chain). FEBS Lett 1988; 241:136-140.

63. Baba T, Watanabe K, Kashiwabara S, Arai Y. Primary structure of human proacrosin deduced from cDNA sequence. FEBS Lett 1989; 244:296-300.

64. Kennedy WP, Polakowski KL. Evidence for an intrazymogen mechanism in the conversion of proacrosin into acrosin. Biochemistry 1981; 20:2240-2245.

65. Jones R, Brown CR, Lancaster T. Carbohydrate-binding properties of boar sperm proacrosin and assessment of its role in sperm-egg recognition and adhesion during fertilization. Development 1988; 102:781-792.

66. Ahuja KK. Carbohydrate determinants involved in mammalian fertilization. Am J Anat 1985; 174:207-223.

67. Huang TTF, Ohzu E, Yanagimachi R. Evidence suggesting that L-fucose is part of the recognition signal for sperm-zona pellucida attachment in mammals. Gamete Res 1982; 5:355-361.

68. Peterson RN, Russell LD, Hunt WP. Evidence for specific binding of uncapacitated boar spermatozoa to porcine zona pellucida in vitro. J Exp Zool 1984; 231:137-147.

69. Huang TTF, Yanagimachi R. Fucoidan inhibits attachment of guinea pig spermatozoa to the zona pellucida through binding to the inner acrosomal membrane and equatorial segment. Exp Cell Res 1984; 153:363-373.

70. Friess AE, Topfer-Petersen E, Schill W-B. Electron microscopic localization of a fucose-binding protein in acrosome-reacted spermatozoa by the fucosyl-peroxidase-gold method. Histochemistry 1987; 86:297-303.

71. O'Rand MG. Inhibition of fertility and sperm zona binding by antiserum to the rabbit sperm membrane autoantigen RSA-1. Biol Reprod 1981; 25:621-628.

72. O'Rand MG, Widren EE, Nikolajczyk BS, Richardson RT, Shabanowitz RB. Receptors for zona pellucida on human spermatozoa. In: Alexander NJ, Griffin PD, Spieler JM, Waites GMH, eds. Gamete Interaction: Prospects for Immunocontraception. New York: Wiley-Liss, 1990:213-226.

73. Herr J, Wright RM, John E, Klotz K, Homyk M, Foster J, Flickinger CJ. Monoclonal antibody MHS-10 and its cognate intra-acrosomal antigen SP-10. In: Alexander NJ, Griffin PD, Spieler JM, Waites GMH, eds. Gamete Interaction: Prospects for Immunocontraception. New York: Wiley-Liss, 1990:13-36.

74. Fulgham DL, Johnson D, Coddington CC, Herr J, Alexander NJ, Hodgen GD. Human sperm acrosome reaction rate on zona pellucida: a time course study. Fertil Steril. In press.

75. Lee GC-Y, Liu M-S, Zhu J-B. Studies of sperm antigens reactive to HS-11 and HS-63 monoclonal antibodies. In: Alexander NJ, Griffin PD, Spieler JM, Waites GMH, eds. Gamete Interaction: Prospects for Immunocontraception. New York: Wiley-Liss, 1990:37-52.

76. Shaha C, Suri A, Talwar GP. Identification of sperm antigens that regulate fertility. Intl J Androl 1988; 11:479-491.

77. Shaha C, Sheshadri TM, Talwar GP, Suri A. Sperm antigens defined from polyclonal antisera. In: Alexander NJ, Griffin PD, Spieler JM, Waites GMH, eds. Gamete Interaction: Prospects for Immunocontraception. New York: Wiley-Liss, 1990:75-88.

78. Benet-Rubinat JM, Martinez P, Andolz P, Garcia-Frams V, Bielsa MS, Egonzcue J. Analysis of human sperm antigens obtained by affinity chromatography with polyclonal antisperm antibodies. J Reprod Immunol 1989(suppl):38.

79. Wang LJ, Miao SY, Liu QY, Bai Y, Xu C, Chen F, Yan YC, Koide S. Antisperm antibodies in sera of chinese infertile subjects and identification of cDNA coding for a specific antigen. J Reprod Immunol 1989(suppl):50.

6

Perspectives in Recombinant Pertussis Toxoid Development

W. Neal Burnette

Amgen Inc.
Thousand Oaks, California

INTRODUCTION

Bordetella pertussis, the etiological agent of whooping cough, was isolated by Jules Bordet in the waning of the Golden Age of classic bacteriology (1). Prophylactic medicine was in its ascendancy and captured the public's imagination through such popular literature as Upton Sinclair's *Arrowsmith* (2) and Paul de Kruif's *The Microbe Hunters* (3). But although vaccines and sera for prevention of infectious diseases proliferated, including toxoids for tetanus and diphtheria, nearly 40 years would pass from Bordet's report in 1906 before a vaccine for pertussis became widely available in the United States (4-7).

Notwithstanding its relatively unrefined composition of whole, chemically inactivated bacterial cells, pertussis vaccine proved strikingly effective for control of whooping cough (8). But as the incidence of disease declined, underlying adverse consequences of pertussis immunization took on greater significance (9-13). The failure of the general public to appreciate the risk-benefit ratio of vaccination is a cautionary tale in preventive medicine; coupled with the emergence of personal-injury litigation as a means for compensating those purportedly injured by "unavoidably unsafe" pharmaceuticals, these phenomena led to a crisis in vaccine confidence (14,15). With regard to pertussis vaccine, the results were a decline in vaccine acceptance, withdrawal of manufacturers from the market, a distressing depletion in the U.S. vaccine reserves, and a consequent increase in disease frequency (8,16).

The paucity of knowledge concerning *B. pertussis* and its pathogenic mechanisms, and its facility to elicit both immunity to disease *and* undesired immunization reactions, prevented any substantial improvement in vaccine safety. The recent application of the tools of molecular biology and protein engineering have brought about a revolution in understanding of pertussis, from which will come newer, safer, and effective vaccines against this fearsome childhood disease. A portion of this research effort is recounted here.

WHOOPING COUGH: DISEASE, EPIDEMIOLOGY, ETIOLOGY, AND CONTROL

The Disease and Its Epidemiology

Whooping cough is a severe respiratory disease with occasionally serious neurological sequelae. It produces its greatest morbidity and mortality in infants less than one year of age (14,17,18). By early in this century, nearly three-fourths of the population of the United States acquired clinical disease by 17 years of age (14,19). Universal vaccination in the United States has reduced the incidence from a high of 265,269 reported cases in 1934 (20), or about 157 cases per 100,000 population (8,21), to less than one case per 100,000 by 1973 (14). As a result of adverse publicity regarding vaccine side effects, acceptance has declined measurably; 3450 cases of whooping cough were reported to the Centers for Disease Control in 1988 (22), although the actual number of infections is believed to be 10- to 20-fold greater (22).

The incidence of whooping cough has likewise registered a substantial decrease in the rest of the developed world where widespread infant vaccination has been employed (8,23-26). However, in the underdeveloped nations of the globe, it has been estimated that 20-60 million cases of pertussis occur each year, resulting in perhaps one million deaths annually (27); thus, a child dies of this vaccine-preventable disease every 30-60 seconds.

The early, or catarrhal, stage of the disease process is characterized by relatively mild coldlike symptoms (28,29). The etiological agent is present during this phase in the nasopharynx and can be controlled by certain antibiotics, such as erythromycin (30-33). Unfortunately, precise diagnosis of early pertussis infection is neither effective nor generally attempted (34-43); differential diagnosis from *Mycoplasma pneumoniae* and adenovirus infections often entails demonstration of lymphocytosis (44). Even in the absence of active or maternal immunity, the infectious organism is eventually cleared from the upper respiratory tract (although it may occasionally be cultured from the lower respiratory tract and from macrophages), but not before leaving behind a residue of toxic constituents at the mucosal epithelium that contribute to the paroxysmal stage of disease (45,46). A major component of this residuum is a complex protein exotoxin, commonly referred to as pertussis toxin (PTX), or pertussigen (47); in fact, whooping cough is considered to be a disease of this toxin (48, 49). Although other pertussis factors, such as the peptidoglycan tracheal cytotoxin (50-54), may contribute synergistically to the coughing spasms associated with severe disease, the systemic manifestations of disease (e.g., hypoglycemia, lymphocytosis, histamine sensitization) and the occasional neurological manifestations appear to be the result of the biological effects of PTX (45).

Bordetella pertussis

The etiological agent of whooping cough is the gram-negative bacillus *B. pertussis* (1). It possesses a number of factors that confer virulence (55), such as PTX (48), adenylate cyclase toxin (56-64), filamentous hemagglutinin (FHA) (65-69), and a dermonecrotic toxin (70-73), all of which appear to be regulated by a bacterial virulence gene *vir* (55,74-76), now called the *bvg* locus (77-80). The aforementioned tracheal cytotoxin appears to damage the ciliated respiratory epithelial cells, resulting in decreased mucociliary activity (53,81). Putative adhesins may contribute to bacterial colonization and ultimate virulence of *B. pertussis*: agglutinogens (82-86) and a 69-kD protein ("pertactin") (87-90); it should be noted that FHA and PTX also function as adhesins (69,91-93).

Infection with *B. pertussis* accords lifelong immunity to disease (19, 94,95). It is nonetheless obscure which bacterial antigens elicit this prolonged protective response; indeed, it is not yet reasonably understood whether protective immunity is provided by humoral or cell-mediated responses, or a combination of both (96-104). For these reasons, many of the bacterial constituents described above have been considered as individual replacements for the whole-cell vaccine. Extensive clinical evaluations of "acellular" component vaccines (see below) nevertheless seem to indicate that PTX is a necessary, if not sufficient, immunogen in vaccines devised to offer protection against severe disease in the neonatal population at greatest risk (105-112).

Control

Chemically inactivated whole-cell vaccines have, for 65 years, demonstrated their clinical effectiveness to provide adequate protective immunity in infants (6,7,24,113-122). The recent development of fractionated acellular vaccines has been an attempt to reduce the high rate of adverse reactions associated with the whole-cell vaccines (9,14,123-149). Although perhaps flawed in their design, numerous clinical trials strongly suggest that such component vaccines may afford an efficacy against severe disease equivalent to that of whole-cell products (105,107-109). The manufacturing processes to produce *Bordetella*-derived antigens are expensive and complex: They necessitate fermentation and operator handling of the human pathogen and extensive purification of relatively minute amounts of product, and still require treatment with formalin or glutaraldehyde to inactivate the biological activities of the main vaccine components (such as PTX) and any contaminating toxic constituents. This latter toxoiding step modifies the structure of the antigens, interferes with their epitopic presentation, and tends to diminish their effective immunogenicity (150-160). The intention of recent research endeavors has been to produce potential vaccine components by recombinant DNA means in heterologous host cells; it was anticipated that this could provide significant quantities of material free from contaminating *B. pertussis* toxic factors. In addition, it was hoped that recombinant means could be found to selectively inactivate the biological effects of the vaccine components without diminishing their immunogenic potential (161). The first target of this research was PTX.

PERTUSSIS TOXIN

Structure

PTX is a hexameric protein with an A-B architecture (Figure 1) similar to that of other related bacterial toxins, such as *Vibrio cholerae* toxin and *Escherichia coli* heat-labile enterotoxin (162-165). The A ("active") protomer of PTX is composed of a single S1 subunit of 26,026 daltons (164,

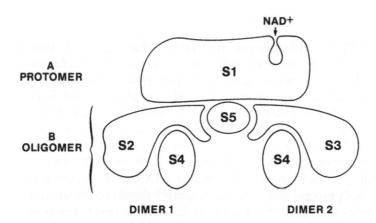

Figure 1 Schematic representation of pertussis toxin. The toxin is hexameric, composed of five different polypeptide subunits. Dimers of S2-S4 and S3-S4 are joined by the S5 subunit to form the B oligomer. Subunits S2 and S4 possess cell receptor recognition sites. The A protomer, or S1 subunit, is enzymatically active: NAD is hydrolyzed to nicotinamide and ADP-ribose, the latter product being transferred to an acceptor substrate involved in cell signal transduction. (From Ref. 332.)

166-169); it is this enzymatic component of the molecule that confers many of its biological activities (170-173). The B ("binding") oligomer is a complex pentamer containing subunits S2 (21,925 d), S3 (21,873 d), S4 (12,059 d) and S5 (11,013 d), in a molar ratio of 1:1:2:1, respectively (164,166). B oligomer acts as the delivery platform for the S1 subunit, contributing cell-receptor recognition functions to the molecule (164,174-178) and permitting it to be internalized through the lipid membrane (92,175,179-183). These adhesin properties reside in the S2 and S3 subunits (92,169,180, 184-188), which share significant amino acid sequence homology (166, 169,189); however, each of these subunits appears to recognize structurally distinct cellular receptors: glycolipid moieties (91,169,190) and glycoproteins for S3 (92,191). It is not apparent how the toxin finds its way out of *B. pertussis*, or where and how it assembles its subunits into the holotoxin form (192-195). Tamura et al. (164) demonstrated that purified PTX could be dissociated into its component subunits and then reassembled in vitro, perhaps in a cooperative and coordinated manner similar to that of cholera toxin (196).

Function

PTX is an ADP-ribosyltransferase (167,168), a characteristic it shares with a number of other bacterial toxins, such as those from *V. cholerae, E. coli, Pseudomonas aeruginosa,* and *Corynebacterium diphtheriae* (197-200). Enzymes of the class possessed by pertussis, cholera, and *E. coli* ADP-ribosylate the α-subunits of certain guanine nucleotide-binding (G) proteins that regulate signal transduction in mammalian cell membranes (201-204). Their activity involves the glycohydrolysis of NAD, the release of nicotinamide and ADP-ribose, and the covalent transfer of the latter moiety to the G protein (198,205-211). PTX appears to have a specificity for the G_i protein that transmits inhibitory signals to the adenylate cyclase complex (212-215); intervention in this transduction pathway disengages control of the synthesis of cyclic AMP, resulting in the cytological effects that give rise to local and systemic toxicity (47,170,172,173,199, 216). A convenient in vitro measure of PTX cytotoxic effects is its ability to provoke a clustered morphology in cultured Chinese hamster ovary (CHO) cells (171,217-219); this assay also provides a sensitive evaluation of the potential toxin-related reactogenicity of pertussis vaccines (113, 218,220-223).

The enzyme-mediated toxicity of PTX has long been known to manifest itself in quantifiable pharmacological effects (224), whence the toxin has acquired a number of synonyms: stimulation of pancreatic islet cells to secrete insulin and produce hypoglycemia (islet-activating protein, or IAP), sensitization to the effects of histamine (histamine-sensitizing factor, or HSF), elicitation of a profound lymphocytosis (lymphocytosis-promoting factor, or LPF), and amplification of immune responses (adjuvanting effect). This panoply of biological activities can be seen in experimental animals given PTX (160,165,172,173,225-250) and, more or less, in vaccinees (251) and in patients with whooping cough (45,160,163,172,173, 240,251-258). It is not yet evident how these consequences of intoxication directly result in the significant symptoms of pertussis. Neither is it explicitly understood how the toxin provokes neurological responses, such as those implicated in the more severe adverse reactions to pertussis vaccine (236,259), although it has been suggested that PTX enhances the permeability of the vascular epithelium and, by this means, causes a breach of the blood-brain barrier (165,260).

Serology

Clinical trials of monocomponent acellular vaccines containing purified, inactivated PTX have demonstrated their distinct effectiveness in the prevention of severe disease. Nonetheless, specific serological correlates of human immunity to pertussis have yet to be unambiguously defined (104, 107,110,113,222,223,261-269). A number of investigations, using both native toxin and recombinant analogs, have mapped humoral epitopes of the S1 subunit (161,270-277). Monoclonal antibodies against the toxin have shown it to possess a number of antigenic determinants capable of eliciting protection in mice against challenge with *B. pertussis* and against various effects of toxin (151,185,188,272,278-281). In one recent study (H. Sato, personal communication), selected monoclonal antibodies against the A protomer and each of the B oligomer subunits, with the exception of S4, exhibited some passive protection in mice against aerosol challenge with *B. pertussis*. The most effective monoclonal antibody, anti-S1 1B7, displayed activity against ADP-ribosyltransferase, against toxin-mediated histamine sensitization and lymphocytosis, and against both aerosol *and* intracerebral challenge of mice with the organism. Active immunization of mice with native B oligomer alone can also elicit aerosol protection (178,186,282), whereas immunization with S1 does not (283). However, the protective epitope(s) of the S1 subunit is dominant in the toxin and seems to improve the protective capabilities of B oligomer (270,272,273, 282,284-289). Because both the A and B components of the toxin appear to possess such immunoprotective determinants, and because the holotoxin is much more immunogenic than its individual elements (perhaps by virtue of its size, insoluble particulate nature, and possible cooperative induction of epitope conformation), the fully assembled toxin molecule would seem to be the most likely vaccine candidate.

Likewise, no correlation between cell-mediated immune responses to PTX and protection against disease has yet been demonstrated (99, 100,263,290). This is an area of intense interest; recent investigations have shed some light on the array, if not the importance, of T-cell epitopes in the toxin and its S1 subunit (99-102,284,285,287,288,290). Chemical toxoiding of PTX could be expected to modify both B- and T-cell epitopes, limiting any relative contributions they might make to protective immunity. We anticipated that rational site-specific alteration of selected amino acid residues in the toxin, by mutagenesis of their codons, could produce a "genetic toxoid" (see discussion below) in which the essential domains of toxicity are irreversibly modified without altering humoral or cellular immune responses. Preliminary results (K. Redhead and K. Mills, personal communication) indicate that chemically detoxified PTX fails to elicit T-cell activation in cultured spleen cells of mice recovering from pertussis lung infection. On the other hand, native PTX, recombinant S1, and an inactive genetic analog of S1 (see below) each stimulate proliferation and IL-2 production, indicative of an antigen-specific T-cell response that is annulled by chemical toxoiding.

MOLECULAR CLONING AND RECOMBINANT EXPRESSION OF PERTUSSIS TOXIN

Molecular Cloning of the Toxin Operon

The pertussis toxin gene was molecularly cloned and sequenced J. M. Keith and his colleagues (166,291) and by R. Rappuoli and co-workers (189). Its structure indicated an operon, with a promoter and a polycistron. The sequence revealed the gene (cistronic) order of the individual PTX subunits: S1, S2, S4, S5, and S3 (Figure 2). The cistronic elements were separated by short intervening sequences, presumably possessing ribosome binding functions. Each gene contained a sequence encoding a putative polypeptide signal sequence, ostensibly for membrane translocation. As previously noted (164), the S4 subunit is synthesized in twice the molar amount of the other individual subunits; the structure of the operon yielded no particular insights into the mechanisms for this phenomenon, although it has been suggested that the S4 gene may somehow be iron-regulated (166).

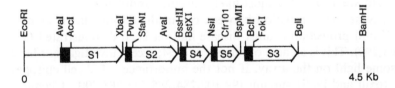

Figure 2   Genetic organization of the pertussis toxin operon. The gene for pertussis toxin was cloned and sequenced (166,291); its organization indicated that it was a polycistronic operon. The figure is a schematic representation of the cistron order (166). The shaded region at the beginning of each cistron denotes its signal sequence. Restriction sites specified were used to subclone each cistronic element into an expression vector. Cloning from just inside the signal sequence, and using the appropriate oligonucleotide linker to restore the open reading frame, resulted in the expression of the full-length preprotein. Cloning just inside the mature open reading frame with an appropriate linker to supply an initiation codon gave the methionyl-mature protein. (From Ref. 283. Reprinted with permission of Nature Publishing Company.)

Recombinant Production of Toxin Subunits in *E. coli*

The individual cistronic elements were subcloned into plasmid vectors for oligonucleotide linker-mediated modifications in preparation for direct, nonfusion expression (283). These modifications included removal of extraneous noncoding sequences from the genes, either retention or removal of the presumed native leader peptide sequences or their substitution with synthetic *E. coli* leader sequences, and the optimal placement of the initiation codon of each gene downstream from a synthetic consensus *E. coli* ribosome binding site. In the case of S1, the native leader sequence was additionally modified by substitution of a serine codon for the single cysteine codon in the leader (166,283) to preclude inappropriate disulfide formation. For expression of mature subunits (i.e., lacking signal peptide sequences), a methionine initiation codon was inserted immediately upstream of that for the putative residue of the mature amino-terminus.

Each gene construct was transferred to plasmid pCFM4722, a vector optimized for high-level direct expression of foreign proteins in *E. coli* under control of an inducible synthetic phage lambda promoter (292). Following transformation of *E. coli*, cell growth, and promoter induction at 42°C, cells were harvested from the fermentation broth and lysed in a French press, and insoluble inclusion bodies were recovered and washed by centrifugation. Each preparation was analyzed by SDS-PAGE (Figure 3), by densitometric scanning of stained gels, and by Western blotting with various polyclonal and monoclonal anti-PTX antibodies.

Subunit S1, expressed with its cysteine-modified signal peptide, was produced as 11.8% of total *E. coli* protein (Table 1); optimization of fermentation conditions has subsequently improved the expression of each of the subunits by substantial levels (unpublished). Essentially all the recombinant S1 protein was found in insoluble inclusions. Under controlled fermentation, the processing of the S1 signal-containing polypeptide to the mature subunit protein was approximately 90% (283). Signal processing of the other subunits was incomplete; substitution of a synthetic, consensus *E. coli* leader for native *B. pertussis* leaders did not improve the proteolytic processing. The recombinant S1, even in its crude form solubilized from inclusions and with no deliberate attempts made to obtain native conformation, was capable of ADP-ribosylating transducin substrate with a specific activity indistinguishable from that of native S1.

Whereas each of the B oligomer subunits could be produced at high levels in the recombinant cells as methionyl-mature polypeptides (i.e., with a methionine residue substituting for the signal peptide sequence), it was interesting to note that S1 could not (Table 1). The amino-terminal

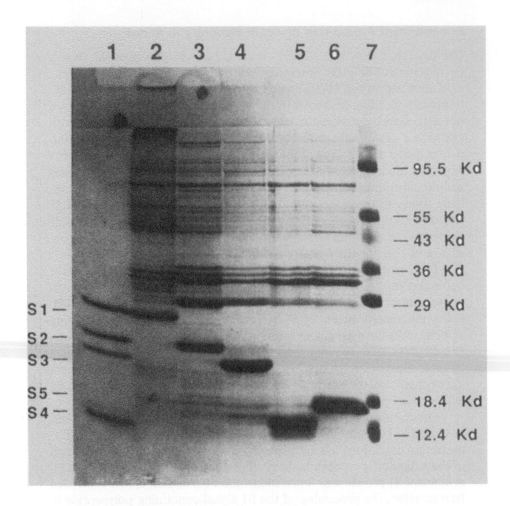

Figure 3 SDS-polyacrylamide gel electrophoresis of recombinant pertussis toxin subunits. *E. coli* transformed with the various expression plasmid constructions were induced at 42°C. Following log-phase growth, the cells were disrupted in a French press and crude inclusion-body pellets obtained by centrifugation of the lysates at 17,000 *g* for 20 minutes. The pellets were subsequently subjected to SDS-PAGE under reducing conditions and the gel stained with Coomassie brilliant blue. Lane 1, native toxin; lane 2, mature recombinant S1; lanes 3, 4, 5, and 6 contain the methionyl-mature species of S2, S3, S4, and S5, respectively; lane 7, molecular weight standards. (From Ref. 332.)

Table 1 Summary of the Expression of Recombinant PTX Subunits in *E. coli*

PTX gene	Plasmid designation	Subunit amino terminus	Extent of signal processing	Level of expression (%)[a]	
				Whole cell	Inclusion bodies[b]
S1	pPTXS1/1	Signal peptide	Complete	11.8	24.8
S1	pPTXS1/2	Methionyl-mature	—	Trace	Trace
S2	pPTXS2/1	Signal peptide	Partial[c]	10.1	11.3
S2	pPTXS2/2	Methionyl-mature	—	1.7	16.8
S3	pPTXS3/1	Signal peptide	None	6.9	20.5
S3	pPTXS3/2	Methionyl-mature	—	4.6	41.3
S4	pPTXS4/1	Signal peptide	NA[d]	Not detectable	Not detectable
S4	pPTXS4/2	Methionyl-mature	—	29.1	49.8
S5	pPTXS5/1	Signal peptide	Partial[c]	21.3[e]	15.9[e]
S5	pPTXS5/2	Methionyl-mature	—	43.8	45.8

[a]Level of expression was obtained by densitometric scanning of Coomassie blue-stained SDS-polyacrylamide gels.
[b]Inclusion bodies were isolated by cell breakage and subsequent low-speed centrifugation.
[c]Percentage of recombinant PTX subunit shown is the sum of the detectable levels of mature, processed subunit and unprocessed preprotein.
[d]Not applicable; no expression could be detected.
[e]Uncorrected for *E. coli* protein contaminates that comigrate in SDS-PAGE with the rPTX subunits.
Source: Ref. 283. Reprinted with permission of Nature Publishing Company.

methionine residues of methionyl-mature S2, S3, and S5 were efficiently removed by the endogenous *E. coli* methionyl aminopeptidase; the amino-terminus of S4 does not contain an amino acid sequence compatible with recognition and cleavage by this enzyme. Expression of each of the PTX subunits with their native primary sequences (with the exception of the methionyl-mature S4) enabled us to conduct structural and functional analyses without the potential obstructions of fusion polypeptides at either end of the molecules. A caveat with the potential to complicate our proposed studies on the complete in vitro assembly of holotoxin from the recombinant subunits (see below) was the contribution, if any, of the individual signal peptide sequences in directing the complex cooperative interactions conceivably involved in the association of native pertussis toxin.

It should also be mentioned that we have attempted to produce all the recombinant subunits in single-cell fermentation by expressing the entire PTX operon, with the signal peptide-encoding sequence of each subunit cistron intact, in *E. coli* (283). In these experiments, the level of subunit production was exceedingly low when compared to the yield of individual subunits expressed under control of the synthetic inducible phage lambda promoter; nor was the expression level significantly enhanced when the phage promoter was substituted for that of the PTX operon promoter. In addition to the problem of signal peptide processing for each of the subunits, as observed for individual expression in *E. coli*, the level of production of each subunit appeared to diminish in direct correlation to relative location of its genetic element in the polycistronic message (283). This latter effect seems to be the result of poor recognition of *B. pertussis*-specific ribosome binding sequences in the intracistronic regions; substitution of the synthetic *E. coli* ribosome binding site for the intervening sequence between the S1 and S2 genes results in amplified expression of the S2 subunit. Although we have continued investigations aimed at the production of all the PTX subunits in single recombinant *E. coli*, it is unlikely that this organism will secrete assembled toxin. Thus, we would still be faced with the need to solubilize intracellular inclusions and reassemble the holotoxin in vitro.

MUTATIONAL MAPPING OF STRUCTURAL CORRELATES OF PERTUSSIS TOXIN FUNCTIONS

Truncation Analysis of the A Protomer

The practical intention of our research efforts was to develop a "genetic" pertussis toxoid—one that lacked the capabilities of reverting to an active form, yet was structurally competent to elicit protective immune responses. The availability of molecular clones of the individual PTX subunit genes (283), prediction of their primary amino acid sequences (166), and the ability to produce these proteins in abundant amounts in recombinant cells (283) permitted us to apply selective site-directed mutagenesis in attempts to modify toxin biochemical and biological activities (271). Of principal concern was the elimination of the enzyme activity from the S1 subunit that contributes to vaccine reactogenicity; secondarily, it would be of interest to alter the cell receptor-recognition characteristics of the B oligomer subunits so as to prevent delivery of the active S1 subunit to sensitive cells while preserving the ability of the toxin to be recognized by appropriate cells of the immune system. A "fail-safe" vaccine might contain a number of mutations in order to disable multiple functional activities and to preclude the remote possibility of genetic reversion to wild-type toxin. However, in the absence of crystallographic data, evaluation of the effects of site-specific modifications on the structure and function of the toxin would necessarily be empirical. For the catalytic S1 subunit, it would be possible to assess the consequences of mutations on its NAD glycohydrolase and ADP-ribosyltransferase activities in vitro. Further, the availability of monoclonal antibodies (188,279-281) would enable detection of changes to the structure of key antigenic determinants.

The S1 subunit can recover its enzymatic activities following extremely harsh treatments, such as boiling in the presence of SDS; this indicates that significant secondary structure is not critical for catalysis. On the other hand, although the passively protective monoclonal antibody 1B7 (which defines the dominant protective epitope of S1) can still *react* with the subunit in a Western blot format after SDS-PAGE (283), the epitope that can *elicit* antibodies of this class is clearly discontinuous and conformational (161,270,271). Thus, a more biological means of analysis would be required to further assess site-specific mutant analogs of S1 that modify its catalytic properties. Because the S1 subunit lacks any detectable biological activity without its association to B oligomer (164,171,175), it would be necessary to achieve assembly of holotoxin with such analogs. Fortunately, the in vitro dissociation-association of native holotoxin had previously been demonstrated (164). The ability of recombinant subunits and their analogs to participate in the coordinated assembly process of holotoxin formation would accomplish at least three objectives: 1) demonstrate their capability to acquire native secondary, tertiary, and quaternary structure, 2) permit evaluation of mutational changes to the toxin for their effects on cultured cells and in vivo, and 3) provide a fully immunogenic holotoxoid that had been inactivated through genetic intervention rather than by chemical modification.

As an adjunct to the cloning and expression of the S1 subunit, two terminally truncated analogs were made (271,275): one that eliminated a portion of the amino terminus (through residue 68) and one that truncated the carboxyl terminus (to residue 187). In preliminary studies, the carboxyl-terminal truncated analog retained both its enzyme activity and its ability to bind monoclonal antibody 1B7; the amino-terminal truncation abolished both of these properties. This suggested that sequences within the first 68 residues of S1 contributed to the formation of a critical enzymatic center and to the organization of the dominant protective epitope. To more precisely map the location of these important domains, the left-hand end of the S1 gene was subjected to limited exonuclease digestion, gene fragments isolated that represented sequential truncations, each inserted into the expression vector with a methionylvaline codon at the translation initiation site, and the encoded polypeptide fragments produced in recombinant *E. coli* (271). After sorting, a representative group of sequence-defined truncated S1 species was selected (Figure 4) and analyzed for NAD glycohydrolase and ADP-ribosyltransferase activity and for reactivity with monoclonal antibody 1B7 and other sera in Western blots.

The results of these analyses (Table 2) show that enzyme activity is retained only by those truncated molecules containing a region from tyrosine-8 through proline-14 (271). Interestingly, this region is one of two major areas of amino acid sequence homology shared among PTX, cholera toxin, and *E. coli* heat-labile enterotoxin (166), the three bacterial ADP-ribosylating toxins having specificity for G proteins. A monoclonal antibody (B2F8) defining the dominant, but nonprotective and nonneutralizing, epitope appears to recognize the sequence amino-terminal to this "homology box" (271,275). Monoclonal antibody 1B7, in addition to its ability to provide passive protection in mice against intracerebral and aerosol challenge, also neutralizes the CHO cell clustering activity and enzyme activities of the toxin (188,280,281). Accordingly, it was not completely unexpected to find that elimination of the homology box by truncation also abolished recognition by this antibody in Western blots (Figure 5).

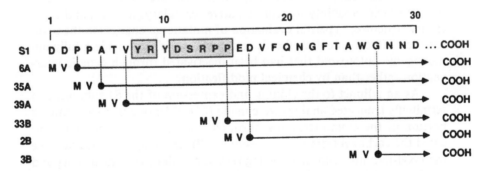

Figure 4 Amino-terminal sequences of truncated S1 proteins. The amino acid sequence of each product was deduced from the DNA sequence. The construction of the expression vectors resulted in the presence of a methionylvaline fusion dipeptide at the beginning of each truncated molecule. The shaded portions of the S1 sequence indicate residue that are identical to those in the homolgous regions of cholera toxin and *E. coli* heat-labile enterotoxin. (From Ref. 271. Reprinted with permission of the National Academy of Sciences.)

Table 2 NAD Glycohydrolase and ADP-Ribosyltransferase Activities of Truncated S1 Proteins

S1 protein	NAD glycohydrolase[a]	ADP-ribosyltransferase[b]
6A	0.85 ± 0.21	26,018 ± 4753
35A	0.87 ± 0.05	5620 ± 771
39A	0.24 ± 0.05	420 ± 177
33B	0.02 ± 0.06	6 ± 10
2B	0.0 ± 0.0	46 ± 80
3B	0.03 ± 0.10	117 ± 203
Purified S1	9.71 ± 0.13	45,839 ± 1662

Values obtained from reactions containing substrate and buffer alone were subtracted from the experimental values prior to calculation.

[a] NAD glycohydrolase activity was determined in samples containing 250 ng of urea-solubilized recombinant S1 or purified S1. Values are the means of triplicate determinations ± standard deviations and are expressed as pmol of nicotinamide released per minute per μg of protein.

[b] ADP-ribosyltransferase activity was determined with 4 μg of purified transducin as substrate and 50 ng of urea-solubilized recombinant S1 or purified S1 as enzyme. Values represent the total acid-precipitable radioactivity (cpm) ± standard deviation, and are the means of triplicate determinations.

Source: Ref. 271. Reprinted with permission of the National Academy of Sciences.

Even if a truncated S1 polypeptide could be folded into a conformation consistent with its incorporation into holotoxin, these findings substantiated that simple deletion of this critical enzymatic center (in order to abrogate reactogenicity of the vaccine material) would result in a toxoid lacking the only recognized protective and neutralizing S1 antigenic determinant.

Site-Directed Mutagenesis and the Toxoiding of the A Protomer

With the available knowledge, the issue remained as to how best to inactivate the S1 subunit without annihilating its ability to acquire a conformation consistent with native presentation of the protective 1B7 epitope and association with B oligomer. In order to more precisely define the contribution of the residues in the homology of box of amino acids 8-14, we set about to modify individual residues in this region by selective site-directed mutagenesis (161). This was accomplished by inserting synthetic oligonucleotides into convenient restriction sites bracketing the homology box. These oligonucleotides contained either single- or double-

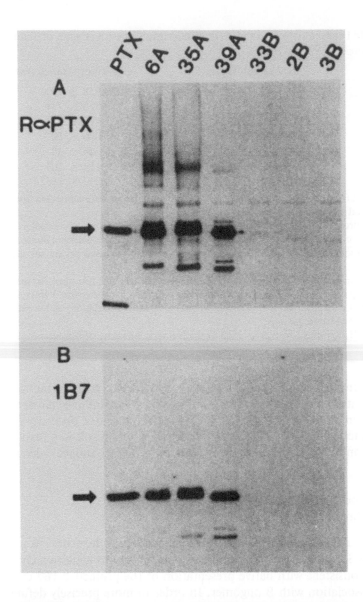

Figure 5 Reaction of recombinant truncated S1 molecules with monoclonal and polyclonal antibodies in Western blots. Aliquots containing equal amounts of recombinant S1 ($\sim 1.0\ \mu$g) or PTX (1.5 μg) were subjected to SDS-PAGE and electrophoretically transferred to nitrocellulose paper (333). Parallel blots were then incubated with either rabbit anti-PTX serum (panel A) or monoclonal antibody 1B7 (panel B). (From Ref. 271. Reprinted with permission of the National Academy of Sciences.)

codon substitutions; they would encode amino acids that would make either conservative or extreme residue substitutions (with respect to charge, relative hydrophobicity, or steric configuration) in the homology box. The initial selection of mutations is shown in Figure 6 and includes a complete deletion of the homology box (161).

Following insertional mutagenesis and expression of the substitution mutants in *E. coli*, the recombinant S1 analogs were again assessed for their enzymatic activities and reactivity with monoclonal antibody 1B7. For convenience of cloning, each of these polypeptide analogs possessed the substitution of methionylvaline for the native amino-terminal aspartylaspartate; this substitution does not result in any significant loss of enzymatic or antigenic activity. Figure 7 reveals that all the single-residue

MUTATION	AMINO-TERMINAL SEQUENCE (1 … 10 … 20 // … 234 COOH)	ACTIVITY: ADP-Ribosyltransferase	ACTIVITY: Neutralizing Epitope
NATIVE	D D P P A T V [Y R] Y [D S R P P] E D V F Q // ··· COOH	+	+
$Y^8 \rightarrow F$	—F— // ··· COOH	+	+
$R^9 \rightarrow K$	—K— // ··· COOH	-	+
$D^{11} \rightarrow E$	—E— // ··· COOH	+	+
$S^{12} \rightarrow G$	—G— // ··· COOH	+	+
$R^{13} \rightarrow K$	—K— // ··· COOH	+	+
$Y^8 \rightarrow L$, $R^9 \rightarrow E$	—L—E— // ··· COOH	-	-
$R^9 \rightarrow N$, $S^{12} \rightarrow G$	—N—G— // ··· COOH	-	-
$D^{11} \rightarrow P$, $P^{14} \rightarrow D$	—P—D— // ··· COOH	-	-
$Y^8 - P^{14}$	—[ ]— // ··· COOH	-	-

Figure 6 Pertussis toxin S1 subunit analog proteins and their activities. The analogs were produced by site-directed mutagenesis of the S1 subunit gene and subsequent expression of the mutated genes in *E. coli.* Oligonucleotide sequencing confirmed the presence of the desired mutation in each analog. The predicted amino acid sequence of the first 20 residues is shown at the top of the figure; the boxed residues comprise the "homology box," as in Figure 4. Mutant Y8-P14 is a deletion of the entire homology region. Enzyme reactivity represents ≥0.02% of the ADP-ribosyltransferase activity of recombinant S1 of native sequence. Reactivity of the epitope represents a discernible response to protective monoclonal antibody 1B7 in Western blots (333). (From Ref. 334.)

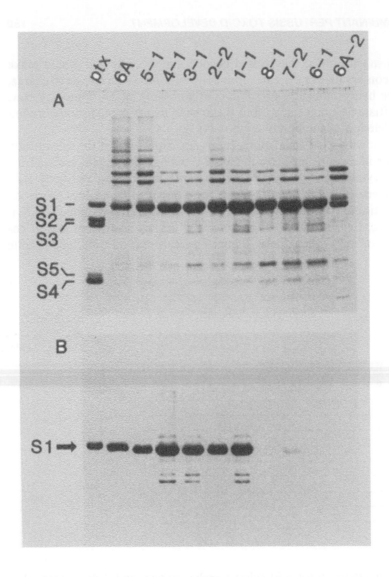

Figure 7 SDS-polyacrylamide gel electrophoresis and Western blot analysis of site-specific mutant S1 proteins. Inclusion body preparations were obtained from recombinant *E. coli* and run in SDS-PAGE. (A) Each S1 mutant preparation (5 μg) and purified PTX (5 μg) was analyzed; the proteins were stained in situ with Coomassie brilliant blue R-250. (B) Each S1 mutant preparation (2.5 μg) and purified PTX (2.5 μg) was analyzed; the proteins were electrophoretically transferred to a nitrocellulose sheet (333) that was subsequently incubated with protective monoclonal antibody 1B7. (From Ref. 161. Reprinted with permission of the American Association for the Advancement of Science.)

mutations preserved the protective epitope, while each of the double mutations abrogated its ability to be formed. When each of the analogs was evaluated for ADP-ribosyltransferase activity, the same general pattern of inactivation was observed; the notable exception was with analog S1/4-1, containing a relatively conservative substitution of lysine for aginine-9 (Table 3). This single amino acid replacement, while conserving the protective epitope, appeared to reduce catalytic activity to negative-control levels. In saturation experiments for ADP-ribosyltransferase, the R9→K analog repeatedly exhibited activity at a level 5000-fold less than native

Table 3 ADP-Ribosyltransferase Activity of Recombinant S1 Mutant Polypeptides

Mutant designation	Amino acid change	Codon change	ADP-ribosyltransferase activity (cpm)
6A	None	None	23,450 ± 950
5-1	Y8→F	TAC→TTC	26,361 ± 1321
4-1	R9→K	CGC→AAG	754 ± 7
3-1	D11→E	GAC→GAA	13,549 ± 1596
2-2	S12→G	TCC→GGC	22,319 ± 2096
1-1	R13→K	CGC→AAG	7393 ± 1367
8-1	Y8→L	TAC→TTG	926 ± 205
	R9→E	CGC→GAA	
7-2	R9→N	CGC→AAC	753 ± 30
	S12→G	TCC→GGC	
6-1	D11→P	GAC→CCG	764 ± 120
	P14→D	CCG→GAC	
20A	Alt. S1 orf	—	839 ± 68

Intracellular inclusions containing the recombinant subunits produced in *E. coli* were recovered by differential centrifugation and extracted with 8 M urea. The urea extracts were adjusted to a total protein concentration of 0.6 mg/ml, dialyzed against 50 mM tris-HCl (pH 8.0), and then centrifuged at 14,000 g for 30 minutes. The amount of recombinant product in the supernatant fractions was determined by quantitative densitometric scanning of proteins separated by SDS-PAGE and stained with Coomassie blue. ADP-ribosyltransferase activity was determined with the use of 4.0 μg of purified bovine transducin and 100 ng of each S1 analog. The values represent the transfer of [^{32}P]-ADP-ribose to the α subunit of transducin, as measured by total trichloroacetic acid-precipitable radioactivity, and each is given as the mean of triplicate determinations with standard deviation. The 20A product, synthesized from a large alternative open reading from within the S1 gene, represents a negative control because its synthesis results in the formation of intracellular inclusions that lack S1-related proteins.
Source: Ref. 271. Reprinted with permission of the American Association for the Advancement of Science.

S1; likewise, little or no NAD glycohydrolase activity could be detected. When the R9→K mutation was introduced into recombinant S1 possessing the native amino-terminal dipeptide sequence (i.e., aspartylaspartate), the resulting analog (S1/1-4) still retained less than 1/1000 of native enzyme activity. Thus, we had created a mutant PTX subunit, toxoided through genetic means rather than by chemical inactivation, with conspicuous potential for use in a pertussis vaccine (161).

Other Structural Correlates of PTX Function

In addition to the seminal observations of S1 structure-function relationships derived through molecular genetic techniques (161,270,271), subsequent studies have provided enlightening detail of antigenic epitopes and enzymatic subsites. As mentioned previously, site-specific mutagenesis and studies with overlapping synthetic peptides have supported biochemical analyses in affording an expositive topography of functional determinants (28,161,164,181-183,270-275,284-286,293-305); in this regard, a key study demonstrated that the dominant protective epitope of the S1 subunit was discontinuous and probably tripartite (270). Another dominant, but nonneutralizing and nonprotective, determinant was shown to contain the free hydrophilic amino terminus (comprising at least residues 1-5) (271,275). Other investigations have focused on defining the enzymatic subsites and critical amino acid residues involved in ADP-ribosyltransferase activity. One such study found that a region bracketing cysteine-41 contributes to features of the S1 subunit important for transferase activity (306); but whereas histidine-35 directly affected catalysis, neither asparagine-34, arginine-39, glutamine-42, nor cysteine-41 itself contributed significantly to enzyme activity. A recent examination of the homology box (residues 8-14) supports a direct role for this region in the binding of the NAD substrate (307).

Of critical importance to an understanding of *B. pertussis* virulence is the recognition of PTX adhesion properties. Both the S2 and S3 subunits, which share considerable amino acid sequence homology, have been implicated in the ability of the toxin to recognize and bind cellular receptors (169,176,184,185,187,190,191,308). Studies with recombinant S2 and selected mutant analogs of this subunit (E. Tuomanen and K. Saukkonen, personal communication) suggest that it specifically recognizes distinctive glycolipid moieties in various cell types. For example, the cell body and isolated cilia of human tracheal epithelial cells each possess a discrete galactose-containing receptor with affinity for S2. Although the cilia of respiratory cells and membranes of monocytic cells appear to share a distinct lactosylseramide-containing S2 receptor, substitution of lysine for histidine-47 in S2 results in the loss of recognition for the cilia-associated glycolipid, with no effect on the monocyte receptor. Continuing investigations are aimed at localization and definition of the carbohydrate recognition domains of the S2 and S3 adhesin components of PTX.

PRODUCTION OF RECOMBINANT PERTUSSIS HOLOTOXOIDS

Analog S1 Expression in *E. coli* and In Vitro Assembly of Holotoxoid

Preservation of the protective antigenic determinants with aboliton of enzyme activity were the hallmarks we desired in a mutated S1 subunit to be utilized in the production of a genetic toxoid vaccine (Figure 8). An

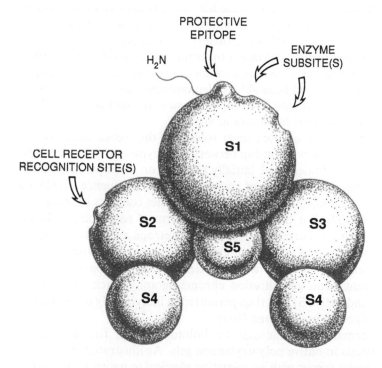

Figure 8 Schematic representation of pertussis toxin. The general position of sequences contributing to the formation of the dominant S1 protective epitope and of a critical catalytic subsite are displayed. (From Ref. 334.)

additional attribute was necessary: the competence of such an analog to acquire a conformation consistent with assembly into the highly immunogenic holotoxin. In the absence of biophysical parameters defining native S1 conformation, such as CD-ORD spectra or crystallographic data, it would be necessary to achieve holotoxin formation in vitro to assess whether S1 could obtain its native structure. Further, in vivo and cell-culture evaluation of the effects of the enzyme-inactivating mutation would require the transport and receptor-recognition functions contributed by the B oligomer subunits.

To this end, we sought to assemble holotoxin in vitro from its component recombinant subunits. On first reflection, this would seem a daunting exercise: Five distinct subunits would need to be folded into an approximation of their native secondary structures following solubilization from *E. coli* inclusion bodies and the quaternary holotoxin formed from these by a possibly tortuous series of cooperative events not replicatable in vitro. Previous experience with the less complex cholera toxin molecule also suggested that the coordinate interactions of its subunits lead to its spontaneous assembly (196); nevertheless, a prerequisite to oligomerization was the appropriate oxidation of intrachain disulfide bonds subsequent to solubilization of recombinant inclusion bodies. And fortunately, Tamura et al. (164) had been able to demonstrate that it was possible to dissociate native PTX into its component subunits and sequentially reassemble the hexameric holotoxin in vitro.

In order to establish the proper folding of the recombinant S1 subunit and evaluate the relationship between its enzyme activity and in vitro and in vivo PTX toxicity, we initially centered on attempts to associate the recombinant S1 molecule of native amino acid sequence (S1/1) and the R9→K S1 analog (S1/1-4) with the B oligomer complex isolated from native PTX (309). For this purpose, each form of recombinant S1 was solubilized from isolated inclusions with chaotrope and reducing agent, the reductant removed, and the single disulfide bond permitted to slowly oxidize in air. The proteins were purified to near-homogeneity by cationic exchange and gel filtration chromatography; each recombinant S1 species and native S1 was then permitted to individually associate with native B oligomer in 2 M urea (309).

The formation of holotoxin (or holotoxoid) was first assessed by electrophoresis in native polyacrylamide gels. As illustrated in Figure 9, macromolecular species with gel migration identical to native PTX could be distinguish in each preparation (309); quantitative densitometric scanning of these gels revealed that oligomerization was very efficient. These results indicated that not only could recombinant S1 be folded into a relatively

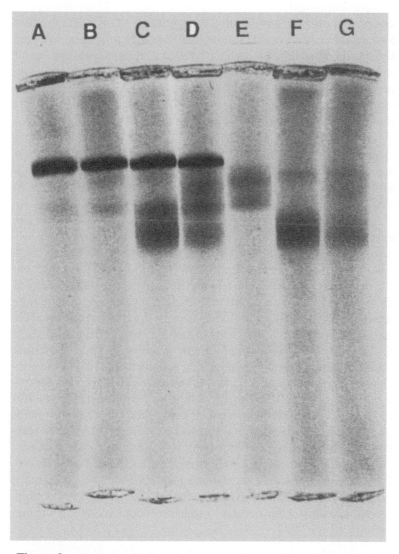

Figure 9 Analysis of holotoxin formation by nondenaturing, nonreducing polyacrylamide gel electrophoresis. Following electrophoresis, proteins in the cylindrical gels were stained with Coomassie brilliant blue R-250. Lanes: (A) 7.5 μg PTX; (B) 2 μg of rS1/1 (recombinant S1 of native amino acid sequence) plus 5.5 μg of B oligomer; (C) 2 μg of rS1/1-4 (recombinant analog S1 of R9→K form) plus 5.5 μg of B oligomer; (D) 2 μg of native S1 plus 5.5 μg of B oligomer; (E) 5.5 μg of B oligomer; (F) 2 μg of rS1/1; (G) 2 μg of rS1/1-4. (From Ref. 309. Reprinted with permission of the National Academy of Sciences.)

native conformation from a disordered state, but that the R9→K mutation had no appreciable affect on the folding and assembly processes. We next evaluated the ability of each preparation to elicit a clustered morphological response in cultured CHO cells (217-219), a cytopathic effect requiring both the enzymatic activity of the S1 subunit and the cell adhesin properties of the B oligomer (171). The results shown in Figure 10 demonstrate that none of the S1 subunit species alone is capable of producing cytotoxicity, that holotoxin formed with recombinant S1 of authentic amino acid sequence (S1/1) evokes a CHO cell clustering response with a specific activity indiscriminate from native PTX, and that the inactive S1 analog-containing holotoxoid lacks the in vitro effect representative of PTX in vivo toxicity.

To measure any residual in vivo toxicity in the holotoxoid species, mice were injected with equivalent doses of either the deactivated S1-containing molecule (S1/1-4 + B oligomer) or native PTX (J. Arciniega and D. Burns, personal communication). Whereas mice injected with native PTX exhibited elevated leukocyte levels, as expected, mice receiving the holotoxoid had leukocyte counts essentially equivalent to those of buffer-injected animals. Moreover, while all mice in the group receiving PTX were sensitized to the lethal effects of histamine, none of the animals in the holotoxoid-injected group were found to be sensitive. Thus, the leukocytosis-promoting and histamine-sensitizing activities of PTX, representative of its in vivo toxicity, directly correlate to in vitro CHO cell clustering activity and to the ADP-ribosyltransferase activity of its S1 subunit.

The totality of the findings described above reinforce the notion that the toxic reactions associated with PTX, and most likely the adverse reactogenicity of incompletely inactivated whole-cell and acellular vaccines, can be attributed to the catalytic effects of the S1 subunit (161,276,296, 309). They also demonstrate that a genetically deactivated S1, produced by recombinant means, can substitute for native S1 in the holotoxin molecule to provide a nonreactive pertussis vaccine component. At this writing,

---

Figure 10 CHO cell clustering activity of holotoxin species assembled in vitro. The samples and their concentrations are as follows: (A) buffer control; (B) B oligomer alone (200 ng/ml); (C) native PTX S1 subunit (50 ng/ml); (D) native PTX (25 ng/ml); (E) enzymatically active rS1/1 alone (50 ng/ml); (F) holotoxin (25 ng/ml) assembled in vitro from native B oligomer and rS1/1; (G) enzymatically inactive rS1/1-4 alone (50 ng/ml); (H) in vitro holotoxin (31.3 ng/ml) composed of native B oligomer and rS1/1-4. (From Ref. 309. Reprinted with permission of the National Academy of Sciences.)

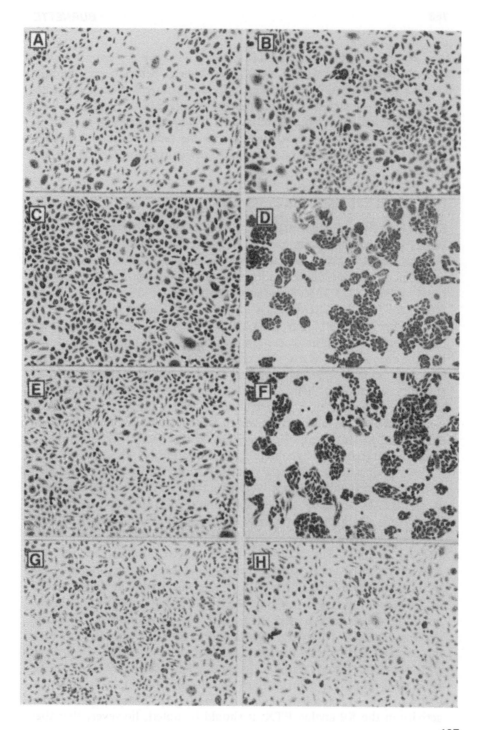

the ''semirecombinant'' holotoxoid (S1/1-4 + native B oligomer) is being compared to chemically toxoided whole-cell pertussis vaccine and native PTX for its ability to protect mice against aerosol challenge with *B. pertussis*. The results of mouse-protection experiments conducted with genetic analogs of *B. pertussis*-derived PTX containing similar mutations in the S1 subunit (see below) suggest that the semirecombinant toxoid with the *E. coli*-produced S1 analog will provide solid protection against challenge.

Holotoxoid Expression in *B. pertussis*

Subsequent to our demonstration of the feasibility of creating a deactivated, yet structurally competent, S1 subunit by selective site-specific mutagenesis (161,271), Klein and his co-workers constructed an extensive series of single- and double-codon substitution mutants in the gene for the S1 subunit (277,310). These substitutions centered on arginine-9 and glutamate-129, the latter predicated upon the apparent participation of this residue in NAD binding (294,298,305). These S1 gene analogs were then inserted into plasmids containing the PTX operon and introduced into the chromosome of tox⁻ *B. pertussis* by homologous recombination. The recombinant organisms were capable of expressing the mutated S1 subunits, assembling them into holotoxin species with the B oligomer subunits, and secreting analog PTX molecules. Not surprisingly, their evaluation of these analogs revealed that the most effective reduction in enzyme activity with retention of the S1 protective epitope was obtained with recombinant toxin species containing S1 mutations R9→K and E129→G.

As a consequence of these results, R. Rappuoli and his colleagues also introduced similar S1 inactivating mutations into the PTX operon of *B. pertussis* by homologous recombination (276,311). The chromosomal S1 cistronic element was replaced with analogs that had been specifically mutagenized at arginine-9 (161), at arginine-13 (161), and/or at glutamate-129 (277,295,305). The mutant PTX analogs were produced and secreted from the recombinant *B. pertussis* genotypes at levels essentially equivalent to those obtained with native PTX. While each of the analogs retained its T-cell and B-cell epitopes, only the R9→K analog and the double mutants (R9→K/E129→G and R13→L/E129→G) exhibited significant decreases in ADP-ribosyltransferase and CHO cell clustering activities; the double mutants were the least active by these criteria. PTX analogs with double mutations were incapable of eliciting leukocytosis or histamine sensitization. In contrast to our results (see above), these investigators were able to detect leukocytosis-promoting and histamine-sensitizing activity in the K9 analog PTX; it should be noted, however, that they utilized doses of the analog 100-fold higher than the median lethal dose of PTX (500 ng per mouse). When evaluated for potency in mice, the double-mutant holotoxoids were capable of providing significant protection against intracerebral challenge with *B. pertussis* in a dose-dependent fashion: Solid immunoprotection was achieved at doses of 4.8-12 μg per animal. These results thus confirmed our findings that selected inactivating mutations in S1 are capable of eliminating the known toxic effects of PTX while retaining its ability to form a holotoxin structure with B oligomer (161,309); moreover, the animal immunoprotective properties of the mutant PTX species prepared by Rappuoli and his co-workers (276,311) affirmed our long-held belief that recombinant toxoid materials may be suitable substitutes for both the whole-cell and acellular pertussis vaccines (161,309).

Progress Toward a Completely Recombinant Pertussis Holotoxoid

B. pertussis has been described as a "dirty little bag of toxins" (312). In addition to PTX, this organism produces adenylate cyclase toxins, tracheal cytotoxin, dermonecrotic toxin, and endotoxins. For this reason, any vaccine product manufactured in *B. pertussis* (regardless of its degree of apparent purity) will, of necessity, need to be chemically treated to eliminate trace contamination by these other toxic pertussis components; such procedures irreversibly modify the antigenic structure of PTX (151,153-155,157,313), reducing its immunoprotective potential and thus negating the advantages achieved through genetic manipulation. The goal of our laboratories has been: 1) to produce a fully recombinant, nonreactogenic, and immunogenic pertussis holotoxoid by biological synthesis in relatively innocuous laboratory strains of *E. coli*, 2) to remove production of the vaccine material from the human pathogen to facilitate operator handling, 3) to obtain the toxoid components at levels of total cell protein that expedite eventual product purity, and 4) to manufacture it by in vitro assembly, enabling precise control of the composition of the final vaccine product.

To this end, we have endeavored to achieve the total in vitro assembly of PTX from all five of the individual recombinant subunits. Expanding on the earlier work of Tamura et al. (164), Sato and colleagues (314) have recently demonstrated the purification of native PTX subunits and their reconstitution into holotoxin. In the interest of manufacturing a cost-effective vaccine material, we have taken a somewhat simpler approach. The individual recombinant subunits are produced in separate *E. coli* fermentations and the insoluble inclusions recovered following cell breakage. These have been mixed in stoichiometric amounts, solubilized in guanidinium hydrochloride under reducing conditions, reoxidized, and permitted to associate by equilibrium dialysis against molar amounts of urea. Preliminary experiments indicate that, with enzymatically active recombinant S1, holotoxin can be formed. As measured by its ability to bind fetuin (164,177,315,316) and to induce CHO cell clustering, this fully recombinant holotoxin is produced with relatively poor efficiency relative to its in vivo assembly in *B. pertussis*. This appears to be the result of the insolubility of the S1 subunit under the laboratory conditions of association.

As an interim solution, we have achieved the efficient in vitro assembly of B oligomer from recombinant subunits S2, S3, S4, and S5. This material can be conveniently purified to near homogeneity, with a suitably low endotoxin content, on fetuin-Sepharose; the quaternary structure possesses the ability to associate with native S1 (unpublished). We are currently evaluating the ability of the recombinant pentamer, minus the S1 subunit, to elicit mouse-protective immune responses. In addition, we are continuing to survey detergent conditions that will increase S1 solubility while still permitting it to associate with the recombinant B oligomer.

HORIZONS IN PERTUSSIS VACCINE DEVELOPMENT

The demand for less reactogenic pertussis vaccines has led to the development of acellular materials for pediatric immunization. These vaccines, composed of more-or-less defined components partially purified from *B. pertussis*, are already in use in Japan; it is anticipated that similar products, primarily containing chemically inactivated PTX, will soon be available in the United States as booster doses for the whole-cell vaccine (317). Recombinant holotoxoid vaccines, with their promise of greater purity, safety, and production control, will constitute the third generation of pertussis vaccines. Of these vaccines manufactured by the techniques of genetic engineering, the genetic toxoid produced in *B. pertussis* is currently in clinical trials (311,318); recombinant toxoid assembled in vitro from *E. coli*-expressed subunits can be expected to eventually supplant *Bordetella*-derived products. As noted earlier, other components of the pertussis bacterium (e.g., FHA, agglutinogens, pertactin) are being investigated as potential vaccine immunogens to augment and amplify the protective responses to PTX.

Discrete PTX subunits, or synthetic peptides representing critical B- and T-cell epitopes of the toxin, may eventually be shown to elicit defined immune responses associated with protection. It is unlikely, however, that such individual antigenic determinants will possess the immunogenic potential of the larger toxin molecule, with its multiple epitopes arrayed in constrained conformations. Of much greater interest, perhaps, is the prospect of using novel recombinant vectors to facilitate the delivery of protective pertussis immunogens. In this regard, heterologous antigen presentation by recombinant vaccinia virus has been demonstrated to stimulate effective humoral and cellular immune responses for a number of viral antigens (319-321). Likewise, oral immunization with recombinant *Salmonella* species expressing foreign antigens can be shown to elicit protective secretory immunity (318,322-324). These recombinant vectors also enjoy the added benefits of providing antigen stability and ease of vaccine administration, particularly in Third World areas where the availability of skilled vaccination personnel, disposable syringes and needles, and cold-chain equipment is severely limited.

The plasma-derived hepatitis B vaccine was probably the last tour de force in the development of human nonrecombinant vaccines (325,326); a few short years saw its replacement with recombinant yeast-derived products of equivalent efficacy (327-331). In efforts to improve their safety, if not their effectiveness, many of the other existing vaccines (e.g., polio, measles, influenza) will inevitably be superseded by recombinant products. Likewise, new vaccines against AIDS, hepatitis C, and malaria will also be produced by genetic engineering techniques. Although whole-cell pertussis vaccine has clearly manifested its ability to control whooping cough in regions of the world where it has been effectively employed, public perception of its hazards has resulted in calls for its improvement. The tools of molecular genetics have now afforded us the means to do so.

ACKNOWLEDGMENTS

I would like to acknowledge the support of Amgen Inc. and the many dedicated colleagues and collaborators who contributed to the studies described herein, especially: J. L. Arciniega, T. D. Bartley, D. L. Burns, K. K. Chen, W. Cieplak, K. T. Kaljot, H. R. Kaslow, J. M. Keith, J. G. Kenimer, K. J. Kim, C. Locht, C. R. Manclark, V. L. Mar, K. S. Marchitto, K. H. G. Mills, C. F. Morris, K. Redhead, R. Sachdev, K. Saukkonen, H. Sato, J. D. Schlotterbeck, R. D. Shahin, R. D. Sublett, E. I. Tuomanen, and D. W. Whiteley.

I also wish to thank the following colleagues, who kindly provided critical reviews of this manuscript: Juan L. Arciniega, Timothy D. Bartley, Drusilla L. Burns, James D. Cherry, Witold Cieplak, Jr., Erik L. Hewlett, Harvey R. Kaslow, Vernon L. Mar, John J. Munoz, Keith Redhead, Hiroko Sato, Roberta D. Shahin, Scott Stibitz, and Elaine Tuomanen.

The work described herein was partly supported at Amgen by grant AI23566-01 and contract AI82679 awarded to the author by the National Institute of Allergy and Infectious Diseases, National Institutes of Health.

REFERENCES

1. Bordet J, Gengou O. Le microbe de la coqueluche. Ann Inst Pasteur 1906; 20:731-741.
2. Sinclair U. Arrowsmith. New York: Harcourt, Brace, 1925.
3. de Kruif P. The Microbe Hunters. New York: Harcourt, Brace, 1926.
4. Kendrick PL, Eldering G. A study in active immunization against pertussis. Am J Hyg 1939; 29:133-153.
5. Felton HM, Willard CY. Current status of prophylaxis by *Hemophilus pertussis* vaccine. J Am Med Assoc 1944; 126:294-299.
6. Kendrick PL. Use of alum-treated pertussis vaccine and of alum-precipitated combined vaccine and diphtheria toxoid for active immunization. Am J Publ Hlth 1942; 32:615-626.
7. Kendrick PL. A field study of alum-precipitated combined pertussis vaccine and diphtheria toxoid for active immunization. Am J Hyg 1943; 38: 193-202.
8. Cherry JD. The epidemiology of pertussis and pertussis immunization in the United Kingdom and the United States: a comparative study. Curr Probl Pediatr 1984; 14:1-78.
9. Hinman AR. DTP vaccine litigation. Am J Dis Child 1986; 140:528-530.
10. Kitch EW. Physicians and the law. Am J Dis Child 1986; 140:525-526.
11. Coulter HL, Fisher BL, DPT: a shot in the dark. New York: Harcourt Brace Jovanovich, 1985.
12. Cherry JD. The controversy about pertussis vaccine. Curr Clin Top Infect Dis 1986; 7:216-238.
13. Yamauchi T. The controversy in clinical medicine regarding the risks and benefits of pertussis immunization. Neurotoxicology 1986; 7:47-52.
14. Cherry JD, Brunell PA, Golden GS, Karzon DT. Report of the task force on pertussis and pertussis immunization—1988. Pediatrics 1988; 81(suppl): 939-984.
15. Peter G. Vaccine crisis: an emerging societal problem. J Infect Dis 1985; 151: 981-983.
16. Bass JW, Stephenson SR. The return of pertussis. Pediatr Infect Dis 1987; 6:141-144.

17. Dauer CC. Reported whooping cough morbidity and mortality in the United States. Publ Hlth Rep 1943; 58:661-676.

18. Centers for Disease Control. Pertussis. Morbid Mortal Weekly Rep 1987; 36:168-171.

19. Gordon JE, Hood RI. Whooping cough and its epidemiological anomalies. Am J Med Sci 1951; 222:333-361.

20. Hinman AR, Koplan JP. Pertussis and pertussis vaccine: reanalysis of benefits, risks, and costs. J Am Med Assoc 1984; 251:3109-3113.

21. Mortimer EA, Jr, Jones PK. An evaluation of pertussis vaccine. Rev Infect Dis 1979; 1:927-934.

22. Centers for Disease Control. Pertussis surveillance—United States, 1986-1988. Morbid Mortal Weekly Rep 1990; 39:57-66.

23. Kanai K. Japan's experience in pertussis epidemiology and vaccination in the past 30 years. Jpn J Med Sci Biol 1980; 33:107-143.

24. Fine PEM, Clarkson JA. Reflections on the efficacy of pertussis vaccines. Rev Infect Dis 1987; 9:866-883.

25. Public Health Service Laboratory. Efficacy of pertussis vaccination in England: report from the PHLS Epidemiological Research Laboratory and 21 area health authorities. Br Med J 1982; 285:357-359.

26. Romanus V, Jonsell R, Bergquist S-O. Pertussis in Sweden after cessation of general immunization in 1979. Pediatr Infect Dis 1987; 6:364-371.

27. Muller AS, Leeuwenburg J, Pratt DS. Pertussis: epidemiology and control. Bull WHO 1986; 64:321-331.

28. Bocka JJ. Pertussis in infants. J Emer Med 1989; 7:345-348.

29. Conway SP, Phillips RR. Morbidity in whooping cough and measles. Arch Dis Child 1989; 64:1442-1445.

30. Bass JW. Erythromycin for treatment and prevention of pertussis. Pediatr Infect Dis 1986; 5:154-157.

31. Bergquist S-O. Erythromycin in the treatment of pertussis. Pediatr Infect Dis 1987; 6:458-461.

32. Bass JW. Use of erythromycin in pertussis outbreaks. Pediatr 1983; 72:748-749.

33. Bass JW, Klenk EL, Kothmeier JB, Linneman CC, Smith MH. Antimicrobial treatment of pertussis. J Pediatr 1969; 75:768-781.

34. Friedman RL, Paulaitis S, McMillan JW. Development of a rapid diagnostic test for pertussis: direct detection of pertussis toxin in respiratory secretions. J Clin Microbiol 1989; 27:2466-2470.

35. Mertsola J, Ruuskanen O, Kuronen T, Meurman O, Viljanen MK. Serologic diagnosis of pertussis: evaluation of pertussis toxin and other antigens in enzyme-linked immunosorbent assay. J Infect Dis 1990; 161:966-971.

36. Onorato IM, Wassilak SGF. Laboratory diagnosis of pertussis: the state of the art. Pediatr Infect Dis 1987; 6:145-151.

37. Campbell PB, Masters PL, Rohwedder E. Whooping cough diagnosis: a clinical evaluation of complementing culture and immunofluorescence with

enzyme-linked immunosorbent assay of pertussis immunoglobulin A in naso-pharyngeal secretions. J Med Microbiol 1988; 27:247-254.

38. Conway SP, Balfour AH, Ross H. Serologic diagnosis of whooping cough by enzyme-linked immunosorbent assay. Pediatr Infect Dis 1988; 7:570-574.

39. Darling WM. Bacteriological diagnosis of pertussis. Lancet 1983; i:246-247.

40. Sotomayor J, Weiner LB, McMillan JA. Inaccurate diagnosis in infants with pertussis. Am J Dis Child 1985; 139:724-727.

41. Preston NW. Recognising whooping cough. Br Med J 1986; 292:901-902.

42. Halperin SA, Bortolussi R, Wort AJ. Evaluation of culture, immunofluor-escence, and serology for the diagnosis of pertussis. J Clin Microbiol 1989; 27:752-757.

43. Centers for Disease Control. Pertussis—Washington, 1984. Morbid Mortal Weekly Rep 1985; 34:390-400.

44. Brooksaler FSW, Buchanan TM. A reappraisal and report of 190 confirmed cases of pertussis. Am J Dis Child 1976; 114:389-396.

45. Pittman M. Neurotoxicity of *Bordetella pertussis*. Neurotoxicol 1986; 7:53-68.

46. Monack D, Munoz JJ, Peacock MG, Black WJ, Falkow S. Expression of pertussis toxin correlates with pathogenesis in *Bordetella* species. J Infect Dis 1989; 159:205-210.

47. Munoz JJ. Biological activities of pertussigen (pertussis toxin). In: Sekura RD, Moss J, Vaughan M, eds. Pertussis Toxin. London: Academic Press, 1985:1-18.

48. Pittman M. The concept of pertussis as a toxin-mediated disease. Pediatr Infect Dis 1984; 3:467-486.

49. Pittman M. Pertussis toxin: the cause of the harmful effects and prolonged immunity of whooping cough. A hypothesis. Rev Infect Dis 1979; 1:401-412.

50. Goldman WE, Klapper DG, Baseman JB. Detection, isolation, and analysis of a released *Bordetella pertussis* product toxic to cultured tracheal cells. Infect Immun 1982; 36:782-794.

51. Goldman WE. *Bordetella pertussis* tracheal cytotoxin: damage to the respir-atory epithelium. In: Schlessinger D, ed. Microbiology—1986. Washington, DC: American Society for Microbiology, 1986:65-69.

52. Cookson BT, Tyler AN, Goldman WE. Primary structure of the peptido-glycan-derived tracheal cytotoxin of *Bordetella pertussis*. Biochemistry 1989; 28:1744-1749.

53. Cookson BT, Cho H-L, Herwaldt LA, Goldman WE. Biological activities and chemical composition of purified tracheal cytotoxin of *Bordetella per-tussis*. Infect Immun 1989; 57:2223-2229.

54. Folkening WJ, Nogami W, Martin SA, Rosenthal RS. Structure of *Borde-tella pertussis* peptidoglycan. J Bacteriol 1987; 169:4223-4227.

55. Weiss AA, Hewlett EL. Virulence factors of *Bordetella pertussis*. Ann Rev Microbiol 1986; 40:661-686.

56. Hewlett EL, Urban MA, Manclark CR, Wolff J. Extracytoplasmic adenylate cyclase of *Bordetella pertussis*. Proc Natl Acad Sci USA 1976; 73:1926-1930.

57. Hewlett EL, Wolff J. Soluble adenylate cyclase from the culture medium of *Bordetella pertussis*: purification and characterization. J Bacteriol 1976; 127: 890-898.

58. Hanski E. Invasive adenylate cyclase toxin of *Bordetella pertussis*. TIBS 1989; 14:459-463.

59. Hanski E, Farfel Z. *Bordetella pertussis* invasive adenylate cyclase: partial resolution and properties of its cellular penetration. J Biol Chem 1985; 290: 5526-5532.

60. Friedman E, Farfel Z, Hanski E. The invasive adenylate cyclase of *Bordetella pertussis*: properties and penetration kinetics. Biochem J 1987; 243: 145-151.

61. Farfel Z, Friedman E, Hanski E. The invasive adenylate cyclase of *Bordetella pertussis*: intracellular localization and kinetics of penetration into various cells. Biochem J 1987; 243:153-158.

62. Monneron A, Ladant D, d'Alayer J, Bellalou J, Bârzu O, Ullmann A. Immunological relatedness between *Bordetella pertussis* and rat brain adenylyl cyclases. Biochemistry 1988; 27:536-539.

63. Ladant D, Brezin C, Alonso J-M, Crenon I, Guiso N. *Bordetalla pertussis* adenylate cyclase: purification, characterization, and radioimmunoassay. J Biol Chem 1986; 261:16264-16269.

64. Gilboa-Ron A, Rogel A, Hanski E. *Bordetella pertussis* adenylate cyclase inactivation by the host cell. Biochem J 1989; 262:25-31.

65. Arai H, Sato Y. Separation and characterization of two distinct hemagglutinins contained in purified leukocytosis-promoting factor from *Bordetella pertussis*. Biochim Biophys Acta 1976; 444:765-782.

66. Brown DR, Parker CD. Cloning of the filamentous hemagglutinin of *Bordetella pertussis* and expression in *Escherichia coli*. Infect Immun 1987; 55: 154-161.

67. Tuomanen E. *Bordetella pertussis* adhesins. In: Wardlaw AC, Parton R, eds. Pathogenesis and Immunity in Pertussis. Chichester, England: John Wiley, 1988:75-94.

68. Tuomanen E. Piracy of adhesins: attachment of superinfection pathogens to respiratory cilia by secreted adhesins of *Bordetella pertussis*. Infect Immun 1986; 54:905-908.

69. Tuomanen E, Weiss A. Characterization of two adhesins of *Bordetella pertussis* for human ciliated respiratory-epithelial cells. J Infect Dis 1985; 152:118-125.

70. Cowell JL, Hewlett EL, Manclark CR. Intracellular localization of the dermonecrotic toxin of *Bordetella pertussis*. Infect Immunol 1979; 25:896-901.

71. Livey I, Wardlaw AC. Production and properties of *Bordetella pertussis* heat-labile toxin. J Med Microbiol 1984; 17:91-103.

72. Bordet J, Gengou O, L'endotoxine coquelucheuse. Ann Inst Pasteur 1909; 23:415-419.

73. Banerjea A, Munoz J. Antigens of *Bordetella pertussis*. II. Purification of heat-labile toxin. J Bacteriol 1962; 84:269-274.

74. Weiss AA, Hewlett EL, Myers GA, Falkow S. Tn5-induced mutations affecting virulence factors of *Bordetella pertussis*. Infect Immun 1983; 42: 33-41.

75. Weiss AA, Melton AR, Walker KE, Andraos-Selim C, Meidl JJ. Use of the promoter fusion transposon Tn5 *lac* to identify mutations in *Bordetella pertussis vir*-regulated genes. Infect Immun 1989; 57:2674-2682.

76. Miller JF, Mekalanos JJ, Falkow S. Coordinate regulation and sensory transduction in the control of bacterial virulence. Science 1989; 243:916-922.

77. Knapp S, Mekalanos JJ. Two *trans*-acting regulatory genes (*vir* and *mod*) control antigenic modulation in *Bordetella pertussis*. J Bacteriol 1988; 171: 5059-5066.

78. Stibitz S, Weiss AA, Falkow S. Genetic analysis of a region of the *Bordetella pertussis* chromosome encoding filamentous hemagglutinin and the pleiotropic regulatory locus *vir*. J Bacteriol 1988; 170:2904-2913.

79. Roy CR, Miller JF, Falkow S. The *bvgA* gene of *Bordetella pertussis* encodes a transcriptional activator required for coordinate regulation of several virulence genes. J Bacteriol 1989; 171:6338-6344.

80. Miller JF, Roy CR, Falkow S. Analysis of *Bordetella pertussis* virulence gene regulation by use of transcriptional fusions in *Escherichia coli*. J Bacteriol 1989; 171:6345-6348.

81. Goldman WE. Tracheal cytotoxin of *Bordetella pertussis*. In: Wardlaw AC, Parton R, eds. Pathogenesis and Immunity in Pertussis. Chichester, England: John Wiley, 1988:231-246.

82. Andersen EK. Serological studies on *H. pertussis, H. parapertussis,* and *H. bronchisepticus*. Acta Pathol Microbiol Scand 1953; 33:202-224.

83. Eldering G, Hornbeck C, Baker J. Serological study of *Bordetella pertussis* and related species. J Bacteriol 1957; 74:133-136.

84. Preston NW, Surapatana N, Carter EJ. A reappraisal of serotype factors 4, 5 and 6 of *Bordetella pertussis*. J Hyg Camb 1982; 88:39-46.

85. Preston NW, Stanbridge TN. Efficacy of pertussis vaccines: a brighter horizon. Br Med J 1972; 3:448-451.

86. Ashworth LAE, Irons LI, Dowsett AB. The antigenic relationship between serotype specific agglutinogens and fimbriae of *Bordetella pertussis*. Infect Immun 1982; 37:1278-1281.

87. Montaraz JA, Novotny P, Ivanyi J. Identification of a 68-kilodalton protective protein antigen from *Bordetella bronchiseptica*. Infect Immun 1985; 47:744-751.

88. Charles IG, Dougan G, Pickard D, et al. Molecular cloning and characterization of protective outer membrane protein P.69 from *Bordetella pertussis*. Proc Natl Acad Sci USA 1989; 86:3554-3558.

89. Brennan MJ, Li ZM, Cowell JL, et al. Identification of a 69-kilodalton non-fimbrial protein as an agglutinogen of *Bordetella pertussis*. Infect Immun 1988; 56:3189-3195.

90. Shahin RD, Brennan MJ, Li ZM, Meade BD, Manclark CR. Characterization of the protective capacity and immunogenicity of the 69-kD outer membrane protein of *Bordetella pertussis*. J Exp Med 1990; 171:63-73.

91. Tuomanen E, Towbin H, Rosenfelder G, et al. Receptor analogs and monoclonal antibodies that inhibit adherence of *Bordetella pertussis* to human ciliated respiratory epithelial cells. J Exp Med 1988; 168:267-277.

92. Brennan MJ, David JL, Kenimer JG, Manclark CR. Lectin-like binding of pertussis toxin to a 165-kilodalton Chinese hamster ovary cell glycoprotein. J Biol Chem 1988; 263:4895-4899.

93. Tuomanen E, Weiss A, Rich R, Zak F, Zak O. Filamentous hemagglutinin and pertussis toxin promote adherence of *Bordetella pertussis* to cilia. Dev Biol Stand 1985; 61:197-204.

94. Hinman AR, Wassilak SFG, Bart KJ. Pertussis. In: Last J, ed. Maxcy-Rosenau Public Health and Preventive Medicine. Vol. 12. Norwalk, CT: Appleton-Century-Crofts, 1986:211-216.

95. Linnemann CC, Jr. Host-parasite interactions in pertussis. In: Manclark CR, Hill JC, eds. International Symposium on Pertussis. DHEW Publ. No. (NIH) 79-1830. Washington, DC: U.S. Government Printing Office, 1979:3-18.

96. Doebbeling BN, Feilmeier ML, Herwaldt LA. Pertussis in an adult man infected with the human immunodeficiency virus. J Infect Dis 1990; 161: 1296-1298.

97. Burstyn DG, Baraff LJ, Peppler MS, Leake RD, StGeme J, Jr, Manclark CR. Serological responses to filamentous hemagglutinin and lymphocytosis-promoting toxin of *Bordetella pertussis*. Infect Immunol 1983; 41:1150-1156.

98. Winsnes R. Serological responses to pertussis. In: Wardlaw AC, Parton R, eds. Pathogenesis and Immunity in Pertussis. Chichester, England: John Wiley, 1988:283-307.

99. Gearing AJH, Bird CR, Redhead K, Thomas M. Human cellular immune responses to *Bordetella pertussis* infection. FEMS Microbiol Immunol 1989; 47:205-212.

100. Gearing AJH, Bird C, Wadha M, Redhead K. The primary and secondary cellular immune responses to whole cell *Bordetella pertussis* vaccine and its components. Clin Exp Immunol 1987; 68:275-281.

101. De Magistris MT, Romano M, Nuti S, Rappuoli R, Tagliabue A. Dissecting human T cell responses against *Bordetella* species. J Exp Med 1988; 168:1351-1362.

102. Fish F, Cowell JL, Manclark CR. Proliferative response of immune mouse T-lymphocytes to the lymphocytosis-promoting factor of *Bordetella pertussis*. Infect Immun 1984; 44:1-6.

103. Granström M, Granström G, Pekka G, Askelöf P. Neutralizing antibodies to pertussis toxin in whooping cough. J Infect Dis 1985; 151:646-649.

104. Zackrisson G, Lagergärd T, Trollfors B. Subclass compositions of immunoglobulin G to pertussis toxin in patients with whooping cough, in healthy individuals, and recipients of a pertussis toxoid vaccine. J Clin Microbiol 1989; 27:1567-1571.

105. Blennow M, Hedenskog S, Granström M. Protective effect of acellular pertussis vaccines. Eur J Clin Microbiol Infect Dis 1988; 7:381-383.

106. Oda M, Higurashi M. Development of acellular pertussis vaccine in Japan. Acta Paediatr Jpn 1988; 30:136-142.

107. Ad Hoc Group for the Study of Pertussis Vaccines. Placebo-controlled trial of two acellular pertussis vaccines in Sweden—protective efficacy and adverse events. Lancet 1988; i:955-960.

108. Olin P. Comparing the efficacy of pertussis vaccines. Lancet 1989; i:95-96.

109. Olin P, Storsaeter J, Romanus V. The efficacy of acellular pertussis vaccines. J Am Med Assoc 1989; 261:560.

110. Robinson A, Irons LI, Ashworth LAE. Pertussis vaccine: present status and future prospects. Vaccine 1985; 3:11-22.

111. Noble GR, Bernier RH, Esber EC, et al. Acellular and whole-cell pertussis vaccines in Japan: report of a visit by US scientists. J Am Med Assoc 1987; 257:1351-1356.

112. Manclark CR, Cowell JL. Pertussis. In: Germanier R, ed. Bacterial Vaccines. New York: Academic Press, 1984:69-106.

113. Griffiths E. Efficacy of whole-cell pertussis vaccine. In: Wardlaw AC, Parton R, eds. Pathogenesis and Immunity in Pertussis. Chichester, England: John Wiley, 1988:353-374.

114. Bell JA. Pertussis prophylaxis with two doses of alum-precipitated vaccine. Publ Hlth Rep Wash 1941; 56:1535-1546.

115. Bell JA. Pertussis immunization: use of two doses of alum-precipiated mixtures of diphtheria toxoid and pertussis vaccine. J Am Med Assoc 1948; 137:1276-1281.

116. Lapin JH. Whooping Cough. Chicago: Charles C Thomas, 1943.

117. Madsen T. Vaccination against whooping cough. J Am Med Assoc 1933; 101:187-188.

118. Madsen T. Whooping cough: its bacteriology, diagnosis, prevention and treatment. Boston Med Surg J 1925; 192:50-60.

119. Medical Research Council. Vaccination Against Whooping Cough: The Final Report to the Whooping Cough Immunization Committee of the Medical Research Council and to the Medical Officers of Health for Battersea and Wandsworth, Bradford, Liverpool and Newcastle. Br Med J 1959; I:994-1000.

120. Sauer LW. Municipal control of whooping cough. J Am Med Assoc 1937; 109:487-488.

121. Blennow M, Olin P, Granström M, Bernier RH. Protective efficacy of a whole cell pertussis vaccine. Br Med J 1988; 296:1570-1572.

122. Jenkinson D. Duration of effectiveness of pertussis vaccine: evidence from a 10 year community study. Br Med J 1988; 296:612-614.

123. Griffith AH. Pertussis vaccines and permanent brain damage. Vaccine 1989; 7:489-490.

124. Miller DL, Wadsworth MJH, Ross EM. Pertussis vaccine and severe acute neurological illnesses. Vaccine 1989; 7:487-489.

125. Leviton A. Neurologic sequelae of pertussis immunization—1989. J Child Neurol 1989; 4:311-314.

126. Blennow M, Granström M. Adverse reactions and serologic response to a booster dose of acellular pertussis vaccine in children immunized with acellular or whole-cell vaccine as infants. Pediatrics 1989; 84:62-67.

127. Dyer C. Judge "not satisfied" that whooping cough vaccine causes permanent brain damage. Br Med J 1988; 296:1189-1190.

128. Shields WD, Nielsen C, Buch D, et al. Relationship of pertussis immunization to the onset of neurologic disorders: a retrospective epidemiologic study. J Pediatr 1988; 113:801-805.

129. Koblin BA, Townsend TR, Muñoz A, Onorato I, Wilson M, Polk BF. Response of preterm infants to diphtheria-tetanus-pertussis vaccine. Pediatr Infect Dis 1988; 7:704-711.

130. Walker AM, Jick H, Perera DR, Thompson RS, Knauss TA. Diphtheria-tetanus-pertussis immunization and sudden infant death syndrome. Am J Publ Hlth 1987; 77:945-951.

131. Walker AM, Jick H, Perera DR, Knauss TA, Thompson RS. Neurologic events following diphtheria-tetanus-pertussis immunization. Pediatrics 1988; 81:345-349.

132. Hoffman HJ, Hunter JC, Damus K, et al. Diphtheria-tetanus-pertussis immunization and sudden infant death: results of the National Institute of Child Health and Human Development Cooperative Epidemiological Study of Sudden Infant Death Syndrome Risk Factors. Pediatrics 1987; 79:598-611.

133. Blattner RJ, Feigin RD. Diphtheria, pertussis, and tetanus (DTP) immunization local reactions do not predict central nervous system reactions. Pediatrics 1986; 78:1168-1169.

134. Lewis K, Cherry JD, Holroyd HJ, Baker LR, Dudenhoeffer FE, Robinson RG. A double-blind study comparing an acellular pertussis-component DTP vaccine with a whole-cell pertussis-component DTP vaccine in 18-month-old children. Am J Dis Child 1986; 140:872-876.

135. Edwards KM, Lawrence E, Wright PF. Diphtheria, tetanus, and pertussis vaccine: a comparison of the immune response and adverse reactions to conventional and acellular pertussis components. Am J Dis Child 1986; 140:867-871.

136. Granström M, Thorén M, Blennow M, Tiru M, Sato Y. Acellular pertussis vaccine in adults: adverse reactions and immune response. Eur J Clin Microbiol 1987; 6:18-21.

137. Blennow M, Granström M, Olin P, et al. Preliminary data from a clinical trial (phase 2) of an acellular pertussis vaccine, J-NIH-6. Dev Biol Stand 1986; 65:185-190.

138. Pichichero ME, Badgett JT, Rodgers GC, McLinn S, Trevino-Scatterday B, Nelson JD. Acellular pertussis vaccine: immunogenicity and safety of an acellular pertussis vs. a whole cell pertussis vaccine combined with diphtheria and tetanus toxoids as a booster in 18- to 24-month old children. Pediatr Infect Dis 1987; 6:352-363.

139. Anderson EL, Belshe RB, Bartram J. Differences in reactogenicity and antigenicity of acellular and standard pertussis vaccines combined with diphtheria and tetanus in infants. J Infect Dis 1988; 157:731-737.

140. Kimura M, Kuno-Sakai H. Acellular pertussis vaccines and fatal infections. Lancet 1988; i:881-882.

141. Blennow M, Granström M, Jäätmaa E, Olin P. Primary immunization of infants with an acellular pertussis vaccine in a double-blind randomized clinical trial. Pediatrics 1988; 82:293-299.

142. Anderson EL, Belshe RB, Bartram J, et al. Clinical and serologic responses to acellular pertussis vaccine in infants and young children. Am J Dis Child 1987; 141:949-953.

143. Storsaeter J, Olin P, Renemar B, et al. Mortality and morbidity from invasive bacterial infections during a clinical trial of acellular pertussis vaccines in Sweden. Pediatr Infect Dis 1988; 7:637-645.

144. Hinman AR, Onorato IM. Acellular pertussis vaccines. Pediatr Infect Dis 1987; 6:341-343.

145. Pollock TM, Morris J. A 7-year survey of disorders attributed to vaccination in Northwest Thames Region. Lancet 1983; i:753-757.

146. Miller DL, Ross EM, Alderslade R, Bellman MH, Rawson NSB. Pertussis immunization and serious acute neurological illness in children. Br Med J 1981; 282:1595-1599.

147. Alderslade R, Bellman MH, Rawson NSB, Ross EM, Miller DL. The National Childhood Encephalopathy Study. In: Whooping Cough: Reports from the Committee on Safety of Medicines and the Joint Committee on Vaccination and Immunization. London: Department of Health and Social Security, Her Majesty's Stationery Office, 1981:79-154.

148. Cody CL, Baraff LJ, Cherry JD, Marcy SM, Manclark CR. Nature and rates of adverse reactions associated with DPT and DT immunizations in infants and children. Pediatrics 1981; 68:650-660.

149. Griffin MR, Ray WA, Mortimer EA, Fenichel GM, Schaffner W. Risk of seizures and encephalopathy after immunization with the diphtheria-tetanus-pertussis vaccine. J Am Med Assoc 1990; 263:1641-1645.

150. Arya SC, Ashraf SJ, Pathak VP. Glutaraldehyde in whole-cell *Bordetella pertussis* vaccine. Vaccine 1989; 7:486.

151. Munoz JJ, Peacock MG. Role of pertussigen (pertussis toxin) on the mouse protective activity of vaccines made from *Bordetella* species. Microbiol Immunol 1989; 33:341-355.
152. Gupta RK, Sharma SB, Ahuja S, Saxena SN. Effects of elevated temperatures on the opacity and toxicity of pertussis vaccines manufactured with different inactivating agents. Vaccine 1986; 4:185-190.
153. Gupta RK, Sharma SB, Ahuja S, Saxena SN. The effects of different inactivating agents on the potency, toxicity and stability of pertussis vaccine. J Biol Stand 1987; 15:87-98.
154. Gupta RK, Saxena SN, Sharma SB, Ahuja S. Studies on the optimal conditions for inactivation of *Bordetella pertussis* organisms with glutaraldehyde for preparation of a safe and potent pertussis vaccine. Vaccine 1988; 6:491-496.
155. Sekura RD, Zhang Y-L, Roberson R, et al. Clinical, metabolic, and antibody responses of adult volunteers to an investigational vaccine composed of pertussis toxin inactivated by hydrogen peroxide. J Pediatr 1988; 113:806-813.
156. Cameron J. Pertussis vaccine: formalin as preferred detoxifying agent. Lancet 1983; i:880-881.
157. Iida T, Horiuchi Y. The detoxification of *Bordetella pertussis* with glutaraldehyde. J Biol Stand 1987; 15:17-26.
158. Ashworth LAE, Robinson A, Irons LI, Morgan CP, Isaacs D. Antigens in whooping cough vaccine and antibody levels induced by vaccination of children. Lancet 1983; ii:878-881.
159. Linggood FV, Stevens MF, Fulthorpe AJ, Wiowod AJ, Pope CG. The toxoiding of purified diphtheria toxin. Br J Exp Pathol 1963; 44:177-188.
160. Munoz JJ, Arai H, Bergman RK, Sadowski PL. Biological activities of crystalline pertissigen from *Bordetella pertussis*. Infect Immun 1981; 33:820-826.
161. Burnette WN, Cieplak W, Mar VL, Kaljot KT, Sato H, Keith JM. Pertussis toxin S1 mutant with reduced enzyme activity and a conserved protective epitope. Science 1988; 242:72-74.
162. Morse SI, Bray KK. The occurrence and properties of leukocytosis and lymphocytosis-stimulating material in the supernatant fluids of *Bordetella pertussis*. J Exp Med 1969; 129:523-550.
163. Morse SI, Morse JH. Isolation and properties of the leukocytosis and lymphocytosis-promoting factor of *Bordetella pertussis*. J Exp Med 1976; 143:1483-1502.
164. Tamura M, Nogimori K, Murai S, et al. Subunit structure of the islet-activating protein, pertussis toxin, in conformity with the A-B model. Biochemistry 1982; 21:5516-5522.
165. Munoz JJ, Bergman RK. *Bordetella pertussis*: Immunological and Other Biological Activities. New York: Marcel Dekker, 1977:1-235.

166. Locht C, Keith JM. Pertussis toxin gene: nucleotide sequence and genetic organization. Science 1986; 232:1258-1264.

167. Katada T, Ui M. Direct modification of the membrane adenylate cyclase system by islet-activating protein due to ADP-ribosylation of a membrane protein. Proc Natl Acad Sci USA 1982; 79:3129-3133.

168. Katada T, Ui M. ADP ribosylation of the specific membrane protein of C6 cells by islet-activating protein associated with modification of adenylate cyclase activity. J Biol Chem 1982; 257:7210-7216.

169. Capiau C, Petre J, Van Damme J, Puype M, Vandekerckhove J. Protein-chemical analysis of pertussis toxin reveals homology between the subunits S2 and S3, between S1 and the A chains of enterotoxins of *Vibrio cholerae* and *Escherichia coli* and identifies S2 as the haptoglobin-binding subunit. FEBS Lett 1986; 204:336-340.

170. Ui M. The multiple biological activities of pertussis toxin. In: Wardlaw AC, Parton R, eds. Pathogenesis and Immunity in Pertussis. Chichester, England: John Wiley, 1988:121-145.

171. Burns DL, Manclark CR. Role of the A subunit of pertussis toxin in alteration of Chinese hamster ovary cell morphology. Infect Immun 1987; 55: 24-28.

172. Munoz JJ. Action of pertussigen (pertussis toxin) on the host immune system. In: Wardlaw AC, Parton R, eds. Pathogenesis and Immunity in Pertussis. Chichester, England, John Wiley, 1988:173-192.

173. Furman BL, Sidey FM, Smith M. Metabolic disturbances produced by pertussis toxin. In: Wardlaw AC, Parton R, eds. Pathogenesis and Immunity in Pertussis. Chichester, England: John Wiley, 1988:147-172.

174. Irons LI, MacLennan AP. Isolation of the lymphocytosis promoting factor-haemagglutinin of *Bordetella pertussis* by affinity chromatography. Biochim Biophys Acta 1979; 580:175-185.

175. Tamura M, Nogimori K, Yajima M, Ase K. Ui M. A role of the B-oligomer moiety of islet-activating protein, pertussis toxin, in development of the biological effects on intact cells. J Biol Chem 1983; 258:6756-6761.

176. Tyrrell GJ, Peppler MS, Bonnah RA, Clark CG, Chong P, Armstrong GD. Lectinlike properties of pertussis toxin. Infect Immun 1989; 57:1854-1857.

177. Sekura RD, Zhang Y-L, Quentin-Millet M-J. Pertussis toxin: structural elements involved in the interaction with cells. In: Sekura RD, Moss J, Vaughan M, eds. Pertussis Toxin. New York: Academic Press, 1985:45-64.

178. Arciniega JL, Burns DL, Garcia-Ortigoza E, Manclark CR. Immune response to the B oligomer of pertussis toxin. Infect Immun 1987; 55:1132-1136.

179. Armstrong GD, Howard LA, Peppler MS. Use of glycosyltransferases to restore pertussis toxin receptor activity to asialogalactofetuin. J Biol Chem 1988; 263:8677-8684.

180. Montecucco C, Tomasi M, Schiavo G, Rappuoli R. Hydrophobic photo-labeling of pertussis toxin subunits interacting with lipids. FEBS Lett 1986; 194:301-304.

181. Nogimori K, Ito K, Tamura M, Satoh S, Ishii S, Ui M. Chemical modification of islet-activating protein, pertussis toxin. Essential role of free amino groups in its lymphocytosis-promoting activity. Biochim Biophys Acta 1984; 801:220-231.

182. Nogimori K, Tamura M, Yajima M, et al. Dual mechanisms involved in development of diverse biological activities of islet-activating protein, pertussis toxin, as revealed by chemical modification of lysine residues in the toxin molecule. Biochim Biophys Acta 1984; 801:232-243.

183. Nogimori K, Tamura M, Yajima M, Hashimura N, Ishii S, Ui M. Structure-function relationship of islet-activating protein, pertussis toxin: biological activities of hybrid toxins reconstituted from native and methylated subunits. Biochemistry 1986; 25:1355-1363.

184. Schmidt MA, Schmidt W. Inhibition of pertussis toxin binding to model receptors by antipeptide antibodies directed at an antigenic domain of the S2 subunit. Infect Immun 1989; 57:3828-3833.

185. Lang AB, Ganss MT, Cryz SJ, Jr. Monoclonal antibodies that define neutralizing epitopes of pertussis toxin: conformational dependence and epitope mapping. Infect Immun 1989; 57:2660-2665.

186. Hausman SZ, Burns DL, Sickler VC, Manclark CR. Immune response to dimeric subunits of the pertussis toxin B oligomer. Infect Immun 1989; 57:1760-1764.

187. Schmidt MA, Schmidt W, Benz I. Antibodies against synthetic peptides of the pertussis toxin S2 subunit: cross-reaction and inhibition of receptor binding. In: Lerner RA, Ginsberg H, Chanock RM, Brown F, eds. Vaccines '89: Modern Approaches to New Vaccines Including Prevention of AIDS. Cold Spring Harbor, NY: Cold Spring Harbor Laboratory, 1989: 253-258.

188. Sato H, Sato Y, Ito A, Ohishi I. Effect of monoclonal antibody to pertussis toxin on toxin activity. Infect Immun 1987; 55:909-915.

189. Nicosia A, Perugini M, Franzini C, et al. Cloning and sequencing of the pertussis toxin genes: operon structure and gene duplication. Proc Natl Acad Sci USA 1986; 83:4631-4635.

190. Francotte M, Locht C, Feron C, Capiau C, De Wilde M. Monoclonal antibodies specific for pertussis toxin subunits and identification of the haptoglobin-binding site. In: Lerner RA, Ginsberg H, Chanock RM, Brown F, eds. Vaccines '89: Modern Approaches to New Vaccines Including Prevention of AIDS. Cold Spring Harbor, NY: Cold Spring Harbor Laboratory, 1989:243-247.

191. Witvliet MH, Burns DL, Brennan MJ, Poolman JT, Manclark CR. Binding of pertussis toxin to eucaryotic cells and glycoproteins. Infect Immun 1989; 57:3324-3330.

192. Sato Y, Arai H, Suzuki K. Leukocytosis-promoting factor of *Bordetella pertussis*. III. Its identity with protective antigen. Infect Immun 1974; 9: 801-810.

193. Perera VY, Wardlaw AC, Freer JH. Release of pertussis toxin and its interaction with outer-membrane antigens. J Gen Microbiol 1987; 133:2427-2435.

194. Perera VY, Freer JH. Accumulation of a precursor of subunit S1 of pertussis toxin in cell envelopes of *Bordetella pertussis* in response to the membrane perturbant phenethyl alcohol. J Med Microbiol 1987; 23:269-274.

195. Hirst TR. Mechanism of enterotoxin secretion from *Escherichia coli* and *Vibrio cholerae*. In: Lark DL, ed. Protein Carbohydrate Interactions in Biological Systems: The Molecular Biology of Microbial Pathogenicity. London: Academic Press, 1986:415-422.

196. Hardy SJS, Holmgren J, Johansson S, Sanchez J, Hirst TR. Coordinated assembly of multisubunit proteins: oligomerization of bacterial enterotoxins *in vivo* and *in vitro*. Proc Natl Acad Sci USA 1988; 85:7109-7113.

197. Yamamoto T, Nakazawa T, Miyate T, Kaji A, Yokota T. Evolution and structure of two ADP-ribosylating enterotoxins, *Escherichia coli* heat-labile toxin and cholera toxin. FEBS Lett 1984; 169:241-246.

198. Moss J, Stanley SJ, Burns DL, et al. Activation by thiol of the latent NAD glycohydrolase and ADP-ribosyltransferase activities of *Bordetella pertussis* toxin (islet-activating protein). J. Biol Chem 1983; 258:11879-11882.

199. Moss J, Vaughan M. ADP-ribosylation of guanine nucleotide-binding regulatory proteins by bacterial toxins. Adv Enzymol 1988; 61:303-379.

200. Wreggett KA. Bacterial toxins and the role of ADP-ribosylation. J Recept Res 1986; 6:95-126.

201. Ui M. Pertussis toxin as a valuable probe for G-protein involvement in signal transduction. In: Moss J, Vaughan M, eds. ADP-Ribosylating Toxins and G Proteins: Insights into Signal Transduction. Washington, DC: American Society for Microbiology, 1990:45-77.

202. Gilman AG. G proteins: transducers of receptor generated signals. Ann Rev Biochem 1987; 56:615-649.

203. Spiegel AM. Signal transduction by guanine nucleotide binding proteins. Molec Cell Endocrinol 1987; 49:1-16.

204. Stryer L, Bourne HR. G proteins: a family of signal transducers. Ann Rev Cell Biol 1986; 2:391-419.

205. Ui M. G proteins identified as pertussis toxin substrates. In: Naccache PH, ed. G Proteins and Calcium Mobilization. Boca Raton, FL: CRC Press, 1989:1-24.

206. Burns DL, Manclark CR. Adenine nucleotides promote dissociation of pertussis toxin subunits. J Biol Chem 1986; 261:4324-4327.

207. West RE, Jr, Moss J, Vaughan M, Liu T, Liu T-Y. Pertussis toxin-catalyzed ADP-ribosylation of transducin: cysteine 347 is the ADP-ribose acceptor site. J Biol Chem 1985; 260:14428-14430.

208. Lim L-K, Sekura RD, Kaslow HR. Adenine nucleotides directly stimulate pertussis toxin. J Biol Chem 1985; 260:2585-2588.

209. Kaslow HR, Lesikar DD. Sulfhydryl-alkylating reagents inactivate the NAD glycohydrolase activity of pertussis toxin. Biochemistry 1987; 26: 4397-4402.

210. Kaslow HR, Lim L-K, Moss J, Lesikar DD. Structure-function analysis of the activation of pertussis toxin. Biochemistry 1987; 26:123-127.

211. Moss J, Stanley SJ, Watkins PA, et al. Stimulation of the thiol-dependent ADP-ribosyltransferase and NAD glycohydrolase activities of *Bordetella pertussis* toxin by adenine nucleotides, phospholipids, and detergents. Biochemistry 1986; 25:2720-2725.

212. Katada T, Oinuma M, Ui M. Mechanisms for inhibition of the catalytic activity of adenylate cyclase by the guanine nucleotide-binding proteins serving as the substrate of islet-activating protein, pertussis toxin. J Biol Chem 1986; 261:5215-5221.

213. Katada T, Oinuma M, Ui M. Two guanine nucleotide-binding proteins in rat brain serving as the specific substrate of islet-activating protein, pertussis toxin. Interaction of the α-subunits with $\beta\gamma$-subunits in development of their biological activities. J Biol Chem 1986; 261:8182-8191.

214. Katada T, Tamura M, Ui M. The A protomer of islet-activating protein, pertussis toxin, as an active peptide catalyzing ADP-ribosylation of a membrane protein. Arch Biochem Biophys 1983; 224:290-298.

215. Bokoch GM, Kateda T, Northrup JK, Hewlett EL, Gilman AG. Identification of the predominant substrate for ADP-ribosylation by islet activating protein. J Biol Chem 1983; 258:2072-2075.

216. Spiegel AM. G proteins in clinical medicine. Hosp Prac 1988; June 15:93-112.

217. Hewlett EL, Sauer KT, Myers GA, Cowell JL, Guerrant RL. Induction of a novel morphological response in Chinese hamster ovary cells by pertussis toxin. Infect Immun 1983; 40:1198-1203.

218. Gillenius P, Jäätmaa E, Askelöf P, Granström G, Tiru M. The standardization of an assay for pertussis toxin and antitoxin in microplate culture of Chinese hamster ovary cells. J Biol Stand 1985; 13:61-66.

219. Iwasa S, Fujiware H. The quantitative assay of the clustering activity of the lymphocytosis-promoting factor (pertussis toxin) of *Bordetella pertussis* on Chinese hamster ovary (CHO) cells. J Biol Stand 1989; 17:53-64.

220. Chazono M, Yoshida I, Konobe T, Fukai K. The purification and characterization of an acellular pertussis vaccine. J Biol Stand 1988; 16:83-89.

221. Quentin-Millet M-J, Arminjon F, Danve B, Cadoz M, Armand J. Acellular pertussis vaccines: evaluation of reversion in a nude mouse model. J Biol Stand 1988; 16:99-108.

222. Robinson A, Ashworth LAE. Acellular and defined-component vaccines against pertussis. In: Wardlaw AC, Parton R, eds. Pathogenesis and Immunity in Pertussis. Chichester, England: John Wiley, 1988:399-417.

223. Cameron J. Evolution of control testing of pertussis vaccines. In: Wardlaw AC, Parton R, eds. Pathogenesis and Immunity in Pertussis. Chichester, England: John Wiley, 1988:419-450.

224. Hewlett EL, Cronin MJ, Moss J, Anderson H, Myers GA, Pearson RD. Pertussis toxin: lessons from biological and biochemical effects in different cells. Adv Cyclic Nucl Prot Phos Res 1984; 17:173-182.

225. Allgaier C, Feuerstein TJ, Jackisch R, Hertting G. Islet-activating protein (pertussis toxin) diminishes α_2-adrenoceptor mediated effects on noradrenaline release. Naunyn-Schmiedeberg Arch Pharmacol 1985; 331:235-239.

226. Araki Y, Yoshida T, Nakamura N, et al. Effect of islet-activating protein (IAP) upon insulin secretion from human islets. Endocrinol Jpn 1981; 28:139-143.

227. Garcia-Sainz JA, Torner ML. Rat fat cells have three types of adenosine receptors (R_p and P). Differential effects of pertussis toxin. Biochem J 1985; 232:439-443.

228. Hewlett EL, Roberts CO, Wolff J, Manclark CR. Biphasic effect of pertussis vaccine on serum insulin in mice. Infect Immun 1983; 41:137-144.

229. Katada T, Ui M. Perfusion of the pancreas isolated from pertussis-sensitized rats: potentiation of insulin secretory responses due to β-adrenergic stimulation. Endocrinology 1977; 101:1247-1255.

230. Katada T, Ui M. Slow interaction of islet-activating protein with pancreatic islets during primary culture to cause reversal of α-adrenergic inhibition of insulin secretion. J Biol Chem 1980; 255:9580-9588.

231. Lai R, Watanabe Y, Yoshida H. Effects of islet-activating protein (IAP) on contractile responses of rat vas deferens: evidence for participation of Ni (inhibitory GTP binding regulating protein) in the α_2-adrenoceptor-mediated response. Eur J Pharmacol 1983; 90:453-456.

232. Parfentjev IA, Schleyer WL. The influence of histamine on the sugar level of normal and sensitized mice. Arch Biochem 1949; 20:341-346.

233. Seino Y, Seino S, Tsuda K, Kuzuya H, Imura H. Islets-activating protein from *Bordetella pertussis*: enhancement of pancreatic somatostatin release. Horm Metabol Res 1983; 15:563-564.

234. Sewell WA, Munoz JJ, Scollay R, Vadas MA. Studies on the mechanism of the enhancement of delayed-type hypersensitivity by pertussigen. J Immunol 1984; 133:1716-1722.

235. Sidey FM, Wardlaw AC, Furman BL. Hypoglycaemia and acute stress-induced hyperinsulinemia in *B. pertussis* infected or pertussis toxin treated mice. J Endocrinol 1987; 112:113-122.

236. Steinman L, Sriram S, Adelman NE, Zanvil S, McDevitt HO, Urich H. Murine model for pertussis vaccine encephalopathy: linkage to H-2. Nature 1982; 299:739-740.

237. Sumi T, Ui M. Potentiation of the adrenergic beta-receptor mediated insulin secretion in pertussis-sensitized rats. Endocrinology 1975; 97:352-358.

238. Yajima M, Hosoda K, Kanbayashi Y, et al. Islet-activating protein (IAP) in *Bordetella pertussis* that potentiates insulin secretory responses of rats. Purification and characterization. J Biochem 1978; 83:295-303.

239. Sato Y, Sato H. Animal models of pertussis. In: Wardlaw AC, Parton R, eds. Pathogenesis and Immunity in Pertussis. Chichester, England, John Wiley, 1988:309-325.

240. Morse SI. Studies on the lymphocytosis induced in mice by *Bordetella pertussis*. J Exp Med 1965; 121:49-68.

241. Wardlaw AC, Parton R. *Bordetella pertussis* toxins. Pharmacol Ther 1983; 19:1-53.

242. Greenberg L, Fleming DS. Increased efficiency of diphtheria toxoid when combined with pertussis vaccine: preliminary note. Can J Publ Hlth 1947; 38:279-282.

243. Lee JM, Olitzky PK. Simple method for enhancing development of acute disseminated encephalomyelitis in mice. Proc Soc Exp Biol Med 1955; 89: 263-266.

244. Munoz JJ, Bernard CCA, Mackay IR. Elicitation of experimental allergic encephalomyelitis (EAE) in mice with the aid of pertussigen. Cell Immunol 1983; 83:92-100.

245. Kong AS, Morse SI. The *in vitro* effects of *Bordetella pertussis* lymphocytosis-promoting factor on murine lymphocytes. I. Proliferative response. J Exp Med 1977; 145:151-162.

246. Kong AS, Morse SI. The *in vitro* effects of *Bordetella pertussis* lymphocytosis-promoting factor on murine lymphocytes. II. Nature of the responding cells. J Exp Med 1977; 145:163-174.

247. Meade BD, Kind PD, Ewell JB, McGrath PP, Manclark CR. *In vitro* inhibition of murine macrophage migration by *Bordetella pertussis* lymphocytosis-promoting factor. Infect Immun 1984; 45:718-725.

248. Meade BD, Kind PD, Manclark CR. Altered mononuclear phagocyte functions in mice treated with the lymphocytosis promoting factor of *Bordetella pertussis*. Dev Biol Stand 1985; 61:63-74.

249. Cortés JMG, Juliano Y, Mendes NF, Mendes E. Delayed type hypersensitivity induced by LPF from *Bordetella pertussis*. Allergol Immunopathol 1986; 14:311-317.

250. Yajima M, Hosoda K, Kanbayashi Y, Nakamura T, Takahashi I, Ui M. Biological properties of islets-activating protein (IAP) purified from the culture medium of *Bordetella pertussis*. J Biochem 1978; 83:305-312.

251. Hannik CA, Cohen H. Changes in plasma insulin concentrations and temperature of infants after pertussis vaccination. In: Manclark CR, Hill JC, eds. International Symposium on Pertussis. DHEW Publ. No. (NIH) 79-1830. Washington, DC: U.S. Government Printing Office, 1979:297-299.

252. Badr-El-Din MK, Aref GH, Mazloum H, et al. The beta-adrenergic receptors in pertussis. J Trop Med Hyg 1976; 79:213-217.

253. Dhar HL, Dhirwani MK, Shethe UK. Pertussis vaccine in diabetes requiring high dose insulin. Br J Clin Prac 1975; 29:119.

254. Furman BL, McMillan M. Does *B. pertussis* vaccine increase insulin secretion by antagonism of endogenous catecholamines? Br J Pharmacol 1985; 84:12P.

255. Regan JC, Tolstoouhov A. Relations of acid base equilibrium to the pathogenesis and treatment of whooping cough. NY State J Med 1936; 36:1075-1087.

256. Toyota T, Kai Y, Kakizaki M, et al. Effects of islet-activating protein (IAP) on blood glucose and plasma insulin in healthy volunteers (Phase I studies). Tohaku J Exp Med 1980; 130:105-116.

257. Walker E, Pinkerton IW, Love WC, Chaudhuri AKR, Datta JB. Whooping cough in Glasgow. J Infect 1981; 3:150-168.

258. Clausen CR, Munoz JJ, Bergman RK. Reaginic-type of antibody in mice stimulated by extracts of *Bordetella pertussis*. J Immunol 1969; 103:768-777.

259. Berg JM. Neurological complications of pertussis immunization. Br Med J 1958; 2:24-27.

260. Amiel SA. The effects of *Bordetella pertussis* vaccination on cerebral vascular permeability. Br J Exp Pathol 1976; 57:653-662.

261. Lau RCH. Pertussis (whooping cough) toxin and *Bordetella pertussis* whole-cell antibody levels in a healthy New Zealand population. NZ Med J 1989; 102:560-562.

262. Thomas MG, Ashworth LAE, Miller E, Lambert HP. Serum IgG, IgA, and IgM responses to pertussis toxin, filamentous hemagglutinin, and agglutinogens 2 and 3 after infection with *Bordetella pertussis* and immunization with whole-cell pertussis vaccine. J Infect Dis 1989; 160:838-845.

263. Wiertz EJHJ, Loggen HG, Walvoort HC, Kreeftenberg JG. *In vitro* induction of antigen specific synthesis and proliferation of T lymphocytes with acellular pertussis vaccines, pertussis toxin and filamentous haemagglutinin in humans. J Biol Stand 1989; 17:181-190.

264. Blennow M, Granström M. Sixteen-month follow-up of antibodies to pertussis toxin after primary immunization with acellular or whole cell vaccine. Pediatr Infect Dis 1989; 8:621-625.

265. Barkin RM, Samuelson JS, Gotlin LP. DTP reactions and serologic response with a reduced dose schedule. J Pediatr 1984; 105:189-194.

266. Manclark CR, Cowell JL. Pertussis vaccine. In: Bell R, Torrigiani C, eds. New Approaches to Vaccine Development. Basel, Switzerland: Schwake, 1984:328-359.

267. Baraff LJ, Leake RD, Burstyn DG, et al. Immunologic response to early and routine DTP immunization in infants. Pediatrics 1984; 73:37-42.

268. Thomas MG, Redhead K, Lambert HP. Human serum antibody responses to *Bordetella pertussis* infections and pertussis vaccination. J Infect Dis 1989; 159:211-218.

269. Redd SC, Rumschlag HS, Biellik RJ, Sanden GN, Reimer CB, Cohen ML. Immunoblot analysis of humoral immune responses following infection with *Bordetella pertussis* or immunization with diphtheria-tetanus-pertussis vaccine. J Clin Microbiol 1988; 26:1373-1377.

270. Bartoloni A, Pizza M, Bigio M, et al. Mapping of a protective epitope of pertussis toxin by *in vitro* refolding of recombinant fragments. Biotechnology 1988; 6:709-712.

271. Cieplak W, Burnette WN, Mar VL, et al. Identification of a region in the S1 subunit of pertussis toxin that is required for enzymatic activity and that contributes to the formation of a neutralizing antigenic determinant. Proc Natl Acad Sci USA 1988; 85:4667-4671.

272. Kaslow HR, Schlotterbeck JD, Kenimer JG. Monoclonal antibodies that inhibit ADP-ribosyltransferase but not NAD-glycohydrolase activity of pertussis toxin. Infect Immun 1990; 58:746-752.

273. Kim JK, Burnette WN, Sublett RD, Manclark CR, Kenimer JG. Epitopes on the S1 subunit of pertussis toxin recognized by monoclonal antibodies. Infect Immun 1989; 57:944-950.

274. Lobet Y, Cieplak W Jr, Smith SG, Keith JM. Effects of mutations on the enzyme activity and immunoreactivity of the S1 subunit of pertussis toxin. Infect Immun 1989; 57:3660-3662.

275. Locht C, Cieplak W, Marchitto KS, Sato H, Keith JM. Activities of complete and truncated forms of pertussis toxin subunits S1 and S2 synthesized by *Escherichia coli*. Infect Immun 1987; 55:2546-2553.

276. Pizza M, Covacci A, Bartoloni A, et al. Mutants of pertussis toxin suitable for vaccine development. Science 1989; 246:497-500.

277. Zealey G, Loosmore S, Cockle S, et al. Construction of *Bordetella pertussis* strains that secrete inactive pertussis toxin analogs. In: Lerner RA, Ginsberg H, Chanock RM, Brown F, eds. Vaccines '89: Modern Approaches to New Vaccines Including Prevention of AIDS. Cold Spring Harbor, NY: Cold Spring Harbor Laboratory, 1989:259-263.

278. Oda M, Cowell JL. Burstyn DG, Thaib S, Manclark CR. Antibodies to *Bordetella pertussis* in human colostrum and their protective activity against aerosol infection of mice. Infect Immun 1985; 47:441-445.

279. Sato H, Sato Y. *Bordetella pertussis* infection in mice: correlation of specific antibodies against two antigens, pertussis toxin, and filamentous hemagglutinin with mouse protectivity in an intracerebral or aerosol challenge system. Infect Immun 1984; 46:415-421.

280. Sato H, Ito A, Chiba J, Sato Y. Monoclonal antibody against pertussis toxin: effect on toxin activity and pertussis infections. Infect Immun 1984; 46:422-428.

281. Kenimer JG, Kim J, Probst PG, Manclark CR, Burstyn DG, Cowell JL. Monoclonal antibodies to pertussis toxin: utilization as probes of toxin function. Hybridoma 1989; 8:37-51.

282. Shahin RD, Simmons M, Manclark CR. Analysis of protection against *Bordetella pertussis* respiratory infection in mice by B oligomer and pertussis toxoid. In: Lerner RA, Ginsberg H, Chanock RM, Brown F, eds. Vaccines '89: Modern Approaches to New Vaccines Including Prevention of AIDS. Cold Spring Harbor, NY: Cold Spring Harbor Laboratory, 1989: 249-252.

283. Burnette WN, Mar VL, Cieplak W, et al. Direct expression of *Bordetella pertussis* toxin subunits to high levels in *Escherichia coli*. Biotechnology 1988; 6:699-706.

284. Kim KJ, McKinness S, Manclark CR. Determination of T cell epitopes on the S1 subunit of pertussis toxin. J Immunol 1990; 144:3529-3534.

285. De Magistris MT, Romano M, Bartoloni A, Rappuoli R, Tagliabue A. Human T cell clones define S1 subunit as the most immunogenic moiety of pertussis toxin and determines its epitope map. J Exp Med 1989; 169:1519-1532.

286. Black WJ, Munoz JJ, Peacock MG, et al. ADP-ribosyltransferase activity of pertussis toxin and immunomodulation by *Bordetella pertussis*. Science 1988; 240:656-659.

287. Oksenberg JR, Ko C, Judd AK, et al. Multiple T and B cell epitopes in the S1 subunit ("A"-monomer) of the pertussis toxin molecule. J Immunol 1989; 143:4227-4231.

288. Oksenberg JR, Judd AK, Ko C, et al. MHC-restricted recognition of immunogenic T cell epitopes of pertussis toxin reveals determinants in man distinct from ADP-ribosylase active site. J Exp Med 1988; 168:1855-1864.

289. Kaslow HR, Schlotterbeck JD, Mar VL, Burnette WN. Recombinant pertussis toxin analogs for vaccine development: neutralizing epitopes of the S1 subunit and enzyme activity. Submitted.

290. Adamson PC, Wu TC, Meade BD, Rubin M, Manclark CR, Pizzo PA. Pertussis in a previously immunized child with human immunodeficiency virus infection. J Pediatr 1989; 115:589-592.

291. Locht C, Barstad PA, Coligan JE, et al. Molecular cloning of pertussis toxin genes. Nucl Acids Res 1986; 14:3251-3261.

292. Morris CF. DNA plasmids. United States Patent 4,710,474 (December 1, 1987).

293. Antoine R, Locht C. Roles of the disulfide bond and the carboxy-terminal region of the S1 subunit in the assembly and biosynthesis of pertussis toxin. Infect Immun 1990; 58:1518-1526.

294. Barbieri JT, Cortina G, ADP-ribosyltransferase mutations in the catalytic S-1 subunit of pertussis toxin. Infect Immun 1988; 56:1934-1941.

295. Cortina G, Barbieri JT. Role of tryptophan 26 in the NAD glycohydrolase reaction of the S-1 subunit of pertussis toxin. J Biol Chem 1989; 264:17322-17328.

296. Pizza M, Bartoloni A, Prugnola A, Silvestri S, Rappuoli R. Subunit S1 of pertussis toxin: mapping of the regions essential for ADP-ribosyltransferase activity. Proc Natl Acad Sci USA 1988; 85:7521-7525.

297. Locht C, Capiau C, Feron C. Identification of amino acid residues essential for the enzymatic activities of pertussis toxin. Proc Natl Acad Sci USA 1989; 86:3075-3079.

298. Barbieri JT, Mende-Mueller LM, Rappuoli R, Collier RJ. Photolabeling of Glu-129 of the S-1 subunit of pertussis toxin with NAD. Infect Immun 1989; 57:3549-3554.

299. Askelöf P, Rodmalm K, Abens J, Undén A, Bartfai T. Use of synthetic peptides to map antigenic sites of *Bordetella pertussis* toxin subunit S1. J Infect Dis 1988; 157:739-742.

300. Edwards KM, Bradley RB, Decker MD, et al. Evaluation of a new highly purified pertussis vaccine in infants and children. J Infect Dis 1989; 160: 832-837.

301. Barbieri JT, Pizza M, Cortina G, Rappuoli R. Biochemical and biological activities of recombinant S1 subunit of pertussis toxin. Infect Immun 1990; 58:999-1003.

302. Burns DL, Hausman SZ, Lindner W, Robey FA, Manclark CR. Structural characterization of pertussis toxin A subunit. J Biol Chem 1987; 262:17677-17682.

303. Presentini R, Perin F, Ancilli G, et al. Studies of the antigenic structure of two cross-reacting proteins, pertussis and cholera toxins, using synthetic peptides. Molec Immunol 1989; 26:95-100.

304. Burns DL, Manclark CR. Role of cysteine 41 of the A subunit of pertussis toxin. J Biol Chem 1989; 264:564-568.

305. Cockle SA. Identification of an active-site residue in subunit S1 of pertussis toxin by photocrosslinking to NAD. FEBS Lett 1989; 249:329-332.

306. Kaslow HR, Schlotterbeck JD, Mar VL, Burnette WN. Alkylation of cysteine 41, but not cysteine 200, decreases the ADP-ribosyltransferase activity of the S1 subunit of pertussis toxin. J Biol Chem 1989; 264:6386-6390.

307. Cieplak W, Jr, Locht C, Mar VL, Burnette WN, Keith JM. Photolabelling of mutant forms of the S1 subunit of pertussis toxin with NAD$^+$. Biochem J 1990; 268:547-551.

308. Schmidt W, Schmidt MA. Mapping of linear B-cell epitopes of the S2 subunit of pertussis toxin. Infect Immun 1989; 57:438-445.

309. Bartley TD, Whiteley DW, Mar VL, Burnette WN. Pertussis holotoxoid formed *in vitro* with a genetically deactivated S1 subunit. Proc Natl Acad Sci USA 1989; 86:8353-8357.

310. Cockle S, Loosmore S, Radika K, et al. Detoxification of pertussis toxin by site-directed mutagenesis. Adv Exp Med Biol 1989; 251:209-214.

311. Nencioni L, Pizza M, Bugnoli M, et al. Characterization of genetically inactivated pertussis toxin mutants: candidates for a new vaccine against whooping cough. Infect Immun 1990; 58:1308-1315.

312. Biotechnology Newswatch 1989; 9:1-3.

313. Larter WE, Corrigan JJ, Fulginiti VA. *In vivo* effect of polymyxin B on pertussis vaccine. Am J Dis Child 1984; 138:281-283.

314. Yamakawa Y, Sato H, Sato Y. Isolation of pertussis toxin subunit proteins by reverse-phase high-performance liquid chromatography and reconstitution of the holotoxin molecule. Anal Biochem 1990; 185:176-181.

315. Sekura RD, Fish F, Manclark CR. Meade B, Zhang Y. Pertussis toxin: affinity purification of a new ADP-ribosyltransferase. J Biol Chem 1983; 258:14647-14651.

316. Chong P, Klein M. Single-step purification of pertussis toxin and its subunits by heat-treated fetuin-sepharose affinity chromatography. Biochem Cell Biol 1989; 67:387-391.

317. Morgan CM, Blumberg DA, Cherry JD, et al. Comparison of acellular and whole-cell pertussis-component DTP vaccines. A multicenter double-blind study in 4- to 6-year-old children. Am J Dis Child 1990; 144:41-45.

318. Moxon ER, Rappuoli R. Modern vaccines: *Haemophilus influenzae* infections and whooping cough. Lancet 1990; 335:1324-1329.

319. Moss B, Smith GL, Mackett M. Use of vaccinia virus as an infectious molecular cloning and expression vector. Gene Amplif Anal 1983; 3:201-213.

320. Moss B, Fuerst TR, Flexner C, Hugin A. Roles of vaccinia virus in the development of new vaccines. Vaccine 1988; 6:161-163.

321. Moss B. Use of vaccinia virus vectors for development of AIDS vaccines. AIDS 1988; 2(suppl 1):S103-S105.

322. Clements JD, El-Morshidy S. Construction of a potential live oral bivalent vaccine for typhoid fever and cholera-*Escherichia coli*-related diarrheas. Infect Immun 1984; 46:564-569.

323. Maskell DK, Sweeney KJ, O'Callaghan D, Hormaeche CE, Liew FY, Dougan G. *Salmonella typhimurium aroA* mutants as carriers of the *Escherichia coli* heat-labile enterotoxin B subunit to the murine secretory and systemic immune systems. Microb Pathogen 1987; 2:211-220.

324. Sadoff JC, Ballou WR, Baron LS, et al. Oral *Salmonella typhimurium* vaccine expressing circumsporozoite protein protects against malaria. Science 1988; 240:236-238.

325. Tite JP, Russell SM, Dougan G, et al. Antivirus immunity induced by recombinant nucleoprotein of influenza A virus. 1. Characteristics and cross-reactivity of T-cell responses. J Immunol 1988; 141:3980-3987.

326. Hilleman MR, Buynak EB, McAleer WJ, McLean AA, Provost PJ, Tytel AA. Newer developments with hepatitis vaccines. Perspect Virol 1981; 11:219-247.

327. Szmuness W, Stevens CE, Harley EJ, et al. Hepatitis B vaccine: demonstration of efficacy in a controlled clinical trial in a high-risk population in the United States. N Engl J Med 1980; 303:832-841.

328. Valenzuela P, Medina A, Rutter WJ, Ammerer G, Hall BD. Synthesis and assembly of hepatitis B surface antigen particles in yeast. Nature 1982; 298: 347-350.

329. Burnette WN, Samal B, Browne J, Bitter GA. Properties and relative immunogenicity of various preparations of recombinant DNA-derived hepatitis B surface antigen. Dev Biol Stand 1985; 59:113-120.

330. Burnette WN, Samal B, Browne JK, Fenton D, Bitter GA. Production of hepatitis B recombinant vaccines. In: Lerner RA, Chanock RM, eds. Modern Approaches to Vaccines: Molecular and Chemical Basis of Virus Virulence and Immunogenicity. Cold Spring Harbor, NY: Cold Spring Harbor Laboratory, 1984:245-250.

331. McAleer WJ, Buynak EB, Maigetter RZ, Wampler DE, Miller DT, Hilleman MR. Human hepatitis B vaccine from recombinant yeast. Nature 1984; 307:178-180.

332. Burnette WN, Mar VL, Cieplak W, et al. Toward development of a recombinant pertussis vaccine. In: Lasky L, ed. Technological Advances in Vaccine Development. New York: Alan R Liss, 1988:75-85.

333. Burnette WN. "Western blotting": electrophoretic transfer of proteins from sodium dodecyl sulfate-polyacrylamide gels to unmodified nitrocellulose and radiographic detection with antibody and radioiodinated protein A. Anal Biochem 1981; 112:195-203.

334. Burnette WN, Bartley TD, Whiteley DW, et al. Recombinant analogs of pertussis toxin S1 subunit. In: Lerner RA, Ginsberg H, Chanock RM, Brown F, eds. Vaccines '89: Modern Approaches to New Vaccines Including Prevention of AIDS. Cold Spring Harbor, NY: Cold Spring Habor Laboratory, 1989:239-242.

VACCINES: CLINICAL AND POLICY DEVELOPMENT

III

7

Vaccine Clinical Trials

John R. La Montagne and George T. Curlin
National Institute of Allergy and Infectious Diseases
National Institutes of Health
Bethesda, Maryland

INTRODUCTION

The widespread availability of vaccines to prevent many of the common infectious diseases of humans has transformed contemporary society. The use of vaccines to prevent disease due to pertussis, measles, mumps, rubella, diphtheria, polio, and tetanus has resulted in massive reductions in the burden of these infections, not only in the United States but throughout the developed world. Dramatic progress has also been achieved in the developing world, where the burden of these infections is most acute. The eradication of smallpox (variola) certainly stands as one of the most important accomplishments, if not *the* most important one, of contemporary medical science. Moreover, polio is now also close to being eradicated in the Western Hemisphere, and it may be eradicated by the end of the decade. Measles, a major killer of children in the world, is another likely candidate for eradication since measles virus has no known reservoir other than humans (1).

Primary prevention of infection by vaccination is extraordinarily effective. It is estimated that the eradication of smallpox results in the savings of approximately $1 billion per year (2). Moreover, and most remarkably, the costs of the eradication program are recovered every 2 months in the United States alone by virtue of the fact that it is no longer necessary to immunize individuals with smallpox vaccine. If these estimates are correct, it means that since variola was eradicated in 1978, approximately $12 billion has been saved! While it is relatively easy to estimate the savings in terms of dollars, the real savings has been in the elimination of smallpox as a cause of disease, death, and disability. As recently as 1974-75, smallpox in India resulted in about 23,500 cases, with a mortality rate of 17.5% (3). These two examples serve as eloquent testimony to the power of vaccines to control disease and save lives.

Despite this astonishing record, vaccine use is at times controversial. This controversy is based almost entirely on concerns about safety (4). There are many reasons for this controversy, but it is due chiefly to two aspects of the use of vaccines. The first is that vaccines are usually used to prevent infectious diseases in normal individuals. Since vaccines are not normally used to treat a disease, the relationship of perceived risk from the vaccine to the perceived benefit from the vaccine must be extremely favorable in the direction of benefit. This means that not only must vaccines be extremely effective in preventing the infection, they must also be extraordinarily safe. The perception of this risk-benefit relationship varies with the disease to prevented. Certainly, during the years when polio was epidemic, the risk of developing paralytic disease from poliovirus infections was readily perceived by the public (5). As a consequence, people were more likely to accept whatever risks were associated with the vaccine in exchange for protection provided by the vaccine.

The second factor in vaccine controversy is that, as vaccines enter common practice, the incidence of infection and disease drops in the community. Consequently, the actual and perceived risk of infection drops. Under these circumstances the perceived risk of adverse events may negatively affect vaccine acceptability. For example, as the use of whole-cell pertussis vaccine increased in the United Kingdom, concerns were raised over the alleged adverse events associated with the use of the whole-cell vaccine, with the ultimate effect of reducing vaccine coverage and eventually leading to severe epidemics of pertussis (7). It has been only in recent years that this situation has been reversed in the United Kingdom, and vaccine acceptability and use have increased.

All these factors lead to the principal focus of this chapter, namely the role of clinical trials in vaccine development. In this chapter we attempt to develop several important themes. The first is that clinical trials are absolutely required for the development and effective use of vaccines. Without well-controlled and well-designed clinical trials, vaccine development would cease. A second important element is that the clinical evaluation of the efficacy and safety of vaccines is a continuing priority, one that must continue even after the vaccines are licensed and in widespread use. Only with this kind of commitment can vaccines themselves be improved, as well as the patterns of vaccine use in the community.

Finally, we are on the threshold of a revolution in biotechnology. This revolution offers the promise that many infectious diseases that are now beyond our ability to control by vaccination, such as malaria or HIV infection, may one day be so controlled. In addition, vaccination greatly enhances the prospect for eradication of infectious diseases. The eradication of smallpox may soon be followed by that of polio and possibly measles. These accomplishments could not have been accomplished without the use and availability of inexpensive vaccines. Finally, vaccines may become available to control or moderate other disease problems. For example, vaccines may be useful in the treatment or prevention of cancer or in the control of fertility in humans, or be used therapeutically to control chronic or persistent infections such as herpes. To achieve these goals it is essential that properly conducted clinical trials be performed, since it is only through the conduct of such trials that the utility of vaccines can be demonstrated.

STEPS IN VACCINE DEVELOPMENT AND THE ROLE OF CLINICAL TRIALS

The development of a vaccine is a multistep process that requires the effective integration of basic and clinical research to be successful. The basic elements required for vaccine development are shown in Table 1. The duration of this process is difficult to estimate for any specific vaccine, as it has been quite variable historically (Table 2). For example, the recent development of an effective hepatitis B vaccine (HBV) required about 40 years from the identification of an etiological agent to the availability of a licensed vaccine (8), while the development of an effective pneumococcal vaccine took almost a century (9). Each case differs, but the ability to move into clinical trials is largely dependent on two factors:

Table 1 Steps in Vaccine Development

I. Basic research
   Identification of causative agent
   Characterization of host's response to infection
   Identification of candidate vaccines
   Development of animal model systems
II. Clinical research
   Phase I, general safety and antigenicity studies
   Phase II, expanded safety and antigenicity studies, to determine optimal dose
      and schedule of immunization
   Phase III, clinical trials to establish efficacy
III. Postlicensure research
   Postmarketing surveillance to confirm safety and efficacy (Phase IV)
   Continued basic and clinical research to develop improved vaccines if necessary

the availability of animal-model systems to study candidate vaccines and the availability of methods to propagate or obtain the causative agent in sufficient amounts to produce candidate vaccines (Table 3). A third factor that confounds these estimates is the availability of alternative approaches to the control of the infectious disease in question. Undeniably, the widespread availability of antibiotics to treat pneumococcal pneumonia after World War II lessened the perceived need to develop pneumococcal vaccines (10).

Table 2 Time Required to Develop Selected Vaccines from Time of Discovery to Licensure

Vaccine	Year agent identified	Year agent propagated	Year vaccine available
Pertussis	1906	1906	1940s
Hepatitis B (plasma)	1940s	1973[a]	1981
Measles	1911	1954	1963
Mumps	1934	1945	1967
Polio	1908	1949	1955
Rubella	1941	1962	1969
Pneumococcal	1881	1881	1977

[a]Year the virus was successfully transmitted to chimpanzees.

Table 3 Major Factors Affecting Vaccine Development

Availability of animal models
Ability to produce antigens in sufficient amounts
Perception that vaccine is necessary for control
Infrastructure for clinical trials

The problems associated with the development of animal-model systems and the production of sufficient amounts of the antigen or antigens are the most important technical obstacles for the development of vaccines. The solution of these problems, however, does not necessarily mean that an effective vaccine can be produced. For example, the etiology of cholera has been known for a century or more, and it has been possible to propagate *Vibrio cholerae* in the laboratory in large amounts for many years. Despite this progress, and the fact that numerous vaccines have been generated and tested to prevent cholera, only in recent years have the bases for effective cholera vaccines become known. These advances required the development of methodology to measure immune responses in the gut. These methods have made it possible to better assess the role of these immune responses and to relate them to protection and to specific *V. cholerae* antigens, such as the toxin (11,12). As a consequence, it is now generally appreciated that gut immunity to several cholera antigens is critical to protection. This has led to the active development of attenuated cholera vaccines and inactivated vaccine preparations that reproducibly appear to confer protective immunity. Similar problems have been noted in the development of vaccines to prevent gonorrhea and other sexually transmitted diseases (STDs) (13).

Finally, it is important to note that a clinical-trial infrastructure is needed if vaccine development is to be successful. The infrastructure and capacity for the basic research in vaccine development are readily available. Moreover, compared to the financial investment required for clinical trials, the costs associated with basic research are lower. It is important, if a promising vaccine candidate is to move effectively down the long path to licensure, that the infrastructure to perform this clinical research be readily available. This is an enormous challenge because clinical research is expensive and, as can be seen from Table 2, the time frame for development is measured in decades, not months or even years. This clinical capability is required to perform the phase I, II, and III research needed to move the vaccine down the developmental path. In the United States, a national system of clinical research centers, the Vaccine Evaluation Units, have been supported by the National Institute of Allergy and Infectious Diseases for almost three decades. It is through these units that much, though certainly not all, of the early phase I and II clinical research on promising new candidate vaccines is performed. Phase III clinical trials, the most expensive single part of the vaccine research effort and often the culmination of long research, often require their own specialized infrastructure and financing. As a consequence, phase III trials often take many years to plan and to perform. The optimal approach for a phase III trial is to establish a dedicated data monitoring and analysis unit to support the trial.

The stepwise progression from basic laboratory studies to clinical investigation to clinical trials outlined above is governed by many factors. Perhaps the single most important factor is the ethical review of vaccine research as it moves into studies in humans. This ethical review will be greatly facilitated by the discovery of new information about the epidemiology, pathogenesis, and host response to infection. Information on these points provides valuable insights into the anticipated effects of a candidate vaccine, including the possibility of adverse events. As clinical studies are initiated, the ethical review focuses primarily on issues concerning safety, although potential benefit is also strongly considered. It is, in fact, these considerations about safety that most dramatically influence vaccine development and research when this research reaches the stage of experimentation in humans.

While it may seem that the development of a vaccine proceeds in a logical manner from laboratory studies to clinical research to licensure, it is important to note that basic and clinical research must continue concurrently. As clinical research progresses, it is critical to incorporate and integrate research findings from these parallel basic research efforts. Only by doing this can unanticipated problems be dealt with effectively. One case in point occurred after the introduction of measles vaccine in 1963 (14). Two vaccines, one attenuated and one killed, were introduced at that time. It was discovered that, while the killed vaccine resulted in atypical measles, vaccinated children became naturally infected. This effect was produced by an aberrant immune response to the inactivated measles virus, a feature that was revealed only by basic research. As a consequence, the killed vaccine was withdrawn from the market.

CLINICAL TRIAL METHODOLOGY

Clinical trials are the most critical process in the development of a vaccine. This process, outlined in Table 4, is conceptualized as a four-stage process. The first stage, phase I, represents the initial efforts to determine that a vaccine candidate is generally safe and antigenic. In this stage the focus is primarily on safety, and the number of experimental subjects in these studies is correspondingly small, usually about 10-15. Phase I vaccine studies are also usually done in individuals at very low risk or no risk of natural infection, and are most effective when done in a double-blind, randomized controlled fashion. This is done to control for intercurrent infection and to maximize the information generated by small numbers of subjects. In certain selected and very specialized situations, phase I studies can be done with the incorporation of an experimental challenge

Table 4 Characteristics of Clinical Phases of Vaccine Research

Phase	Number of subjects	Purpose	Characteristics of study population
I	10-100s	To assess gross safety	Done in populations at low risk to infection Placebo-controlled Double-blind and randomized in design
II	25-1000s	To expand data on safety and to determine optimal dose and schedule	Done in populations at risk to infection Not necessarily placebo-controlled or randomized in design
III	100-10,000s	To establish efficacy and determine safety	Done in populations at risk to infection Usually placebo-controlled, randomized in design
IV	100,000-millions	To confirm safety and efficacy	Population in which vaccine is being used, e.g., children Not randomized Not placebo-controlled Case-control methodology or population-based data often employed

system. Experimental challenge systems in young adult humans are available only for certain respiratory viral pathogens (influenza and rhinoviruses), malaria, and some enteric pathogens. In all these cases, human challenge studies are used because animal-model systems are not faithful models of human infection and the experimental challenge infection in humans is mild or easily treatable. If an experimental challenge infection is possible, additional information on the possible effectiveness of a vaccine can be obtained in a phase I trial.

The demarkation between phase I and phase II trials is often cloudy, but generally after the gross safety and antigenicity of a vaccine have been demonstrated in a phase I trial, efforts ensue to proceed to phase II. In addition to bolstering the data on the safety of the vaccine, the phase II trials are performed to better define dose and schedule of administration. The phase II process can take considerable time and usually involves many more subjects. In certain situations, the movement from phase I to phase II is more complicated. For example, vaccines whose target population are children or infants are subjected to initial phase I studies and perhaps some phase II studies (dose finding) in adults. Only after these are completed is it possible to move on to phase I studies in children and, eventually, infants. In addition to studies in adults, it is often necessary to proceed carefully down in age before clinical studies are performed in infants. The results of these studies must be carefully interpreted because adults, adolescents, and even older children are not faithful immunological surrogates for infants. The infant immune system is still maturing, and the antigenic exposures of adults, adolescents, and older children may confound interpretations of antigenicity or safety. It is because of these factors that it is important to do the phase I and phase II studies in the target population for the vaccine.

In contrast to the phase I trials, phase II trials may not need to be double-blind, placebo-controlled, or randomized in design. However, it should be pointed out that the value added by the double-blind, randomized, and control design is also very great in phase II trials. This is due largely to the risk of intercurrent infection in the population under study and the need to better define the incidence of adverse events to the vaccine. As in the phase I studies, phase II studies are done to determine the optimal schedule of administration and to confirm the safety of the vaccine in the target population. Ultimately, the objective of the phase II trials is to prepare for the phase III clinical trial. Information on dose, schedule, and reactogenicity are critical to the proper design of a phase III trial. Phase II studies may require several hundred to a thousand individuals.

The planning and execution of a phase III trial is a long and complicated process. Unlike the phase I and II studies, the objectives of the phase III trial are to demonstrate the effectiveness of the candidate vaccine in preventing the target disease and to confirm the safety of the vaccine. The planning of a phase III trial requires the interaction of epidemiologists, biostatisticians, clinicians, information specialists, and other scientists, and may take years to complete. Appropriate sites must be identified and the scientific objectives of the trials must be carefully defined. In addition, it is essential to determine that the infrastructure exists to perform the clinical trial. For example, it is important to establish a workable case definition that will be sensitive enough and specific enough to permit the primary endpoint to be achieved. Discussion of and agreement on the secondary endpoints, primarily focused on safety, are also critical.

The favored design for a phase III trial is for a double-blind, placebo-controlled, randomized clinical trial. This represents a "gold standard" that is often not achieved. The feasibility of this kind of trial depends on many factors, but it usually hinges on the acceptability of a placebo control group within the study population. This problem can be dealt with in the design of a clinical trial to some extent by minimizing the size of the control group or by incorporating some form of intervention as the control arm. For example, instead of a saline control group in a trial of acellular pertussis vaccines, the candidate vaccine may be compared to a bivalent tetanus and diphtheria toxoid vaccine.

One salient characteristic of phase III trials is their size. These studies usually involve many thousands of persons and can involve millions. The size factor is one of the major reasons that extreme care must be applied in the planning and execution of such trials, since so much depends on these efforts and it may be extremely difficult to launch similar efforts in the event the trial is unsuccessful. Other approaches to design include assignment of individuals to vaccine or control group by date of birth or by using the nonparticipants as a control arm. These latter options are definitely not optimal in that they introduce biases that are difficult to control and will raise questions about the results obtained that will be impossible to resolve conclusively (15). These options should be entertained only after it is clear that a randomized, double-blind, controlled trial cannot be performed. Finally, some clinical trials are done using case/control methodology. Carefully done clinical trials using case/control methods can be successful (16), but they are usually effective only in circumstances in which the incidence of the disease is low and in which controls can be effectively matched to cases. As with other nonrandom clinical-trial designs, case/control trials are subject to numerous biases that complicate data analyses and cloud the interpretation of these results.

The final phase in vaccine development, so-called phase IV, is the postmarketing assessment of the efficacy and safety of vaccines. This part of the process usually relies on epidemiological investigations of the effect of a vaccine on the population in question. The interpretation of the data from these studies is complicated by the fact that most often case/control methodology is used to assess vaccine efficacy or safety. In addition, phase IV studies may also depend on the passive acquisition of information related to vaccine safety. This is due to the large number of individuals involved in such studies, which may make it necessary to use passive rather than active methods of case ascertainment. More recently, attempts to develop linked data bases as tools in the postmarketing evaluation of vaccines have been explored. Whether the linked data-base systems being established in many communities can be used to answer these questions remains to be determined.

This postmarketing aspect of vaccine development is truly critical. For example, it was through this kind of effort that failure to adequately inactivate poliovirus was determined (17). This led to improvement in the polio vaccine and an increased measure of safety for the public.

RECENT PROGRESS IN VACCINE CLINICAL TRIALS

The revolution in biology that has taken place over the last half century has brought into clinical trial many potential vaccines that were undreamed of fifty years ago. Modern molecular biology and immunology combined with recombinant DNA techniques and the application of monoclonal antibody technology have resulted in many new approaches to vaccine development. Table 5 summarizes some recent developments in vaccine research and development that have occurred within the last three years. Remarkable progress has been made with several vaccines. Seven new vaccines have been approved for use in the United States during the last decade (Table 6). This is a remarkable record in that two of the vaccines—one to prevent hepatitis B virus (HBV) infections, the other to prevent *Haemophilus influenzae* type B (HiB) infections—represent truly new vaccines that were not available before 1980. Perhaps more remarkable is the fact that both the HBV and HiB vaccines have gone from first-generation vaccines to second-generation products in less than one decade. This is particularly encouraging given the problems inherent in performing successful clinical trials in thousands of individuals. It is evidence of the

Table 5 Recent Clinical Trials of Vaccines

Vaccine	Trial design[a]	Phase	Population[b]	n	Location	Ref.	Comments
Acellular pertussis	RS CC, HC	IV	C >2 yr	76	Japan	23	Confirmed efficacy of Japanese acellular vaccines in children >2 years old. However, results are not product-specific since Japanese consider all acellular vaccines similar.
Acellular pertussis	RS CC, HC	IV	C >2 yr	146	Japan	24	Efficacy of acellular pertussis vaccines shown to be approximately 94% in this trial based on a comparison of attack rates of pertussis in siblings of unimmunized children.
Acellular pertussis	D-B, P-C, R	III	C 5-11 yr	3801	Sweden	25	This trial compared the efficacy of vaccines containing only detoxified lymphocytosis-promoting factor (pertussis toxin or LPF) to a vaccine that contained LPF plus filamentous hemagglutinin to placebo. The point efficacy for the LPF vaccine was shown to be about 54 and 69% for the two-component vaccine.

Table 5 Continues

Table 5 Continued

Vaccine	Trial design[a]	Phase	Population[b]	n	Location	Ref.	Comments
HSV-2 subunit glycoprotein	D-B, P-C, R	III	A	161	USA	34	Vaccine failed to protect HSV-2-seronegative sexual partners of HSV-2-positive individuals. Lack or efficacy related to poor immunogenicity of HSV-2 subunit vaccine.
Human gonadotropin + tetanus	M-C	I/II	A(F)	116	India	8	Vaccine stimulated antibody to both tetanus and human gonadotrophin in women who had history of tubal ligation. Antibody titers to both antigens lasted approximately 1 year.
Rhesus rotavirus	D-B, P-C	III	I	200	USA	45	Vaccine induced seroconversion in about 62% of infants; efficacy in preventing rotavirus diarrhea only 38%, presumably due to circulation virus of heterotypic rotavirus in community.
Meningococcal group B		III	A	200,000	Norway	46	Two clinical trials are under way, one in military recruits and the other in

Trial	Design	Phase		N	Location	Ref.	Comments
BCG in leprosy	D-B, P-C, R	III	C + A	5356	PNGᶜ	30	secondary-school students. Final results not yet available. Comparison of BCG to saline in prevention of leprosy in an endemic area. This trial, conducted from 1963 to 1979, demonstrated that BCG provided 48% protection against clinical leprosy and was most effective when used in children <15 years old and against tuberculoid leprosy. There was evidence of accelerated manifestations of tuberculoid leprosy when children <5 years old were immunized.
BCG + killed *M. leprae* vs. BCG	R, not P-C	III	A + C	—	Malawi	32	Ongoing trial comparing repeated doses of BCG alone to BCG + *M. leprae.* The trial is currently under way; results will not be available for several years.
BCG vs. ICRC bacilli	R, not P-C,	III	A + C	—	India	33	Ongoing efficacy trial of ICRC, a mycobacterium that cross-reacts with *M.*

Table 5 Continues

Table 5 Continued

Vaccine	Trial design[a]	Phase	Population[b]	n	Location	Ref.	Comments
							leprae and can induce lepromin conversions in patients with lepromatous leprosy and in lepromin-negative individuals. Study is designed to determine if incidence of leprosy can be reduced in healthy household contacts of leprosy patients.
Oral killed cholera vaccines	R, P-C, D-B	III	C + Ad + F >15 yr	62,285	B[d]	29	Field trial compared the efficacy of killed whole-cell (WC) *Vibrio cholerae* vaccines given orally in protection against cholera as well as non-cholera fibrios (NCV). WC vaccine was given either alone or in combination with purified B subunits. The comparison arm was *E. coli* K12. Both vaccines were effective in preventing cholera, but not in preventing diarrhea due to NCV.

EZ vs. Schwarz measles vaccines	Non-R, not D-B	III	I	GB^e	558	51	Two cohorts of infants were compared; one received the E-Z vaccine (high dose, 40,000 pfu) at 4 months, the second received the standard Schwarz vaccine at 9 months. All cases of measles that occurred during the 2-year follow-up were in the Schwarz vaccine cohort, none in the E-Z cohort.
Mono-JE vs. Bi-JE	R, D-B, P-C	III	C	T^f	65,224	50	Trial compared two Japanese encephalitis (JE) vaccines, a monovalent (Nakayama strain) versus a bivalent (Nakayama plus Beijing strains), versus tetanus toxoid for their ability to prevent JE and/or dengue. Both inactivated JE vaccines were shown to be approximately 95% effective.
HiB PR	CC	IV	C	USA	87,541	47	Multicenter, case/control study of the efficacy of HiB PRP <18 months vaccine performed after the licensure of the PRP

Table 5 Continues

Table 5 Continued

Vaccine	Trial design[a]	Phase	Population[b]	n	Location	Ref.	Comments
							vaccine. The efficacy of the PRP vaccine was estimated to be between 41 and 62% in this nationwide study.
HiB PRP	CC	IV	C	195	USA	48	Case/control study performed in Minnesota. Originally, this <18-month trial was one of the centers in the larger trial (Ref. 14). The point estimate of efficacy derived from this trial was calculated to be approximately 69%. As a consequence of the trial, PRP vaccine was not recommended for use in Minnesota by the state health department.
HiB PRP-D conjugate	R, D-B, P-C	III	C	2102	Alaska	16	Prospective, randomized, placebo-controlled trial performed in Alaska among native-born Alaskan infants. Results indi-

cate that 3 doses of PRP-D (PRP conjugated to diphtheria toxoid) did not protect infants from invasive bacterial disease due to *Haemophilus influenzae*. The estimate of efficacy derived from the trial was calculated to be approximately 31%; moreover, the PRP-D vaccine proved to be poorly immunogenic in this population.

S. typhi Vi	R, D-B, C	III	C + A	6907	Nepal	52	Prospective, double-blind controlled trial of purified Vi polysaccharide vaccine demonstrated that this vaccine was highly effective in preventing typhoid fever in an endemic area.

[a] The following abbreviations are used to describe trial design: R = randomized; P-C = placebo-controlled; D-B = double-blind; HC = household contact; CC = case/control; PS = prospective; and RS = retrospective.
[b] I = infants; C = children; Ad = adolescents; A = adults; F = female.
[c] Papua New Guinea.
[d] Bangladesh.
[e] Guinea-Bissau.
[f] Thailand.

Table 6 Vaccines Introduced into the United
States, 1980-90

Rabies, human diploid	1981
HiB, PRP	1986
HiB, PRP-protein conjugates	1989
HBV (plasma-derived)	1985
HBV (rDNA, produced in yeast)	1987
Attenuated typhoid, Ty21A	1989
Enhanced-potency killed polio	1980

vitality and energy that permeate the vaccine research community. The
other vaccines that entered use represent significant advances in enhancing the antigenicity or improving the safety, or both, of existing vaccine
products. It is likely that the momentum generated during the last decade
will accelerate in the next quarter-century as many of the clinical trials
currently planned or under way are completed.

Major research emphasis has been focused on several important infectious disease problems, including pertussis, AIDS, HiB, cholera, leprosy, herpes, polysaccharide-protein conjugate, and malaria. Research
has also intensified in the development of vaccines that can be used to
control fertility in women or men (8), as well as in the development of
vaccines that can be used for therapeutic purposes, not just prophylacti-
cally (18).

The development of improved pertussis vaccines has been the major
focus of attention for more than a decade (15). The association of adverse
events with the use of the currently licensed and widely used whole-cell
vaccine has been the major driving force in this effort. The liability problems that have emerged from the use of whole-cell pertussis vaccines have
had a very negative impact, particularly on the pharmaceutical industry,
which sees the vaccine component of their product line as a minor, but
very cost-intensive segment (20). It is clear that the liability issues have
been an important stimulus in the development of acellular pertussis vaccines. These vaccines, widely used in Japan to prevent pertussis (21), have
only recently begun the rigorous clinical trials that will be required for
licensure in the United States. Three basic types of acellular pertussis vaccines are under development. All these vaccines are made from cultivated
Bordetella pertussis from which the important antigens have been purified. These antigens include the lymphocytosis promoting factor (LPF,

or pertussis toxin), the filamentous hemagglutinin (FHA), a variety of agglutinogens or fimbriae, and the 69 kD cell surface protein.

Variations on this theme include the generation of nontoxic LPF through recombinant DNA methods (22). These acellular vaccines contain different proportions of LPF to FHA or to the other antigens. Two vaccine types are used in Japan: so called T-type* and B-type (21). Product-specific efficacy data for these vaccines are not available from Japan, although attempts have been made (see Table 5) to document, primarily through case/control studies, the efficacy of the Takeda vaccine (23,24). However, a randomized, double-blind, placebo-controlled trial of a B-type pertussis vaccine was successfully completed in Sweden in 1987 (25). In the Swedish trial, two candidate vaccines were evaluated; one consisted of purified LPF only, the other contained equal amounts of LPF plus FHA. Both vaccines were detoxified with formalin. The efficacy of these two preparations was evaluated in infants more than 6 months of age. Following two doses of vaccine the trial revealed that both products were effective in preventing pertussis in this population, although the efficacy reported (54% for the LPF vaccine and 69% for the LPF:FHA vaccine) was considered low compared to the presumed efficacy of the whole-cell vaccine (15). Newer acellular pertussis vaccines are produced by blending these antigens in varying proportions and adding other bacterial antigens. Among the more interesting acellular pertussis candidates are preparations that include not only LPF and FHA, but the appropriate agglutinogens and the 69kD cell surface protein. A comprehensive phase I/II clinical trial of the 13 available acellular pertussis vaccines is currently under way in the United States. This study is scheduled to be completed by early 1991. It is now projected that at least one phase III trial will be initiated in 1991. The follow-up phase III acellular pertussis trials will differ from the first trial in Sweden in that the vaccine candidates will be administered to infants beginning at 2 months of age, the trial vaccines will also contain diphtheria and tetanus toxoids, and a whole-cell vaccine will be incorporated in one arm of the trial.

The current epidemic of HIV infection has also stimulated a broad-based effort to develop vaccines to prevent this important infection (26). Efforts have been complicated by the fact that HIV is an antigenically variable lentivirus that produces infections that can be latent and lifelong.

---

*T-type refers to vaccines similar to those produced by the Takeda Company. These vaccines contain approximately 90% FHA, 9% LPF, and 1% agglutinogens. In contrast, the B-type vaccines (Biken) contain approximately 50% LPF and 50% FHA.

One of the major impediments has been the absence of an easily manipu-
lated animal-model system. Until recently, only experimental infection
of the chimpanzee was available. However, recent progress with a parallel
model system of simian immunodeficiency virus (SIV) in rhesus monkeys
and the generation of SCID mice reconstituted with human immune cells
will certainly accelerate progress on vaccine candidates (27). Two candidate vaccines have been tested in humans for safety and antigenicity. Both
rely on the use of recombinant DNA technology to produce the surface antigens of HIV. One of these vaccine contains gp160 expressed in insect cells
using baculovirus vectors. The second vaccine employs vaccinia as a vector
for expressing gp160. Clinical studies with both these vaccines continue.

Recent studies in the chimpanzee model suggest that type-specific
protective immunity is possible using gp120, but not gp160 expressed in
chinese hamster ovary (CHO) cells (28). It is certain that these developments will stimulate additional efforts to develop candidate HIV vaccines. However, before clinical trials are performed, many important
problems remain to be resolved. One of the more important questions is
the extent of antigenic variation among HIV viruses. An international
effort to assess the extend of this variation will probably be required.
Perhaps the more difficult question concerns the identification of sites
where efficacy trials can be performed. Almost certainly, trials of efficacy will have to be performed in those regions of the globe where the
risk of infection is high, such as central Africa. The problems inherent
in organizing and conducting such trials represent important challenges,
but the problem is so important that effective ways to evaluate the efficacy of candidate HIV vaccines will be found.

Progress has also been made in the development and testing of vaccines to prevent cholera (29,30) and leprosy (31,32). These two ancient
plagues of mankind have not been amenable in the past to control using
vaccines. In the case of leprosy, though, significant progress has been
made. One clinical trial conducted in the 1960s demonstrated that immunization with BCG had some beneficial effect in preventing leprosy. This
trial has stimulated at least two other phase III clinical trials of vaccines
to prevent leprosy. One trial (32), in Malawi, seeks to compare BCG with
a vaccine containing BCG plus inactivated *Mycobacterium leprae*. Another approach has been to use a cultivatable mycobacterium that apparently possess antigenically cross-reactive components to *M. leprae*
(33). This latter trial is currently under way in India.

In the case of cholera, recent clinical trials have shown the value of
oral immunization with either inactivated or attenuated *Vibrio cholerae*

vaccines. Immune response to the B subunit of the cholera toxin was thought to be important in immunity to cholera, but recent clinical trials indicate that immune response to the B subunit is not important (30). In these studies, oral inactivated vaccines that did not contain the B subunit were just as effective as vaccines that did. Progress has also been made in the development of attenuated cholera vaccines. Several vaccine candidates have been evaluated over the last decade. It appears that protection from infection by *V. cholerae* is determined by immune response to somatic antigens of the vibrio rather than specific immunity to the toxin.

The sexually transmitted diseases (STDs), as a group, represent one category of infectious diseases that have so far eluded efforts at vaccine development. The wide diversity of the organisms responsible for STDs complicates the technical problems associated with the control or prevention of these infections. Not only do STDs represent a major uncontrolled infectious disease problem in the United States, there is growing evidence indicating that STDs are important cofactors that facilitate HIV infections. Both these reasons are powerful arguments to accelerate the development of effective vaccines to prevent STDs. Prevention through vaccination remains an alternative if several technical problems are solved, particularly the stimulation of protective mucosal immunity. While only hepatitis B vaccine is currently available to prevent an STD, efforts are under way to develop vaccines to prevent other STDs. Most notable are efforts to develop vaccines to prevent genital herpes. Vaccines to prevent herpes simplex virus (HSV-1 and HSV-2) infections are actively under development. One of these vaccines, containing purified subunits of HSV-2, was evaluated in sexual partners of HSV-2-infected individuals (34). The vaccine failed to protect the seronegative sexual partners from infection, presumably because of its poor immunogenicity. The development of attenuated HSV-1/HSV-2 vaccine is also under way (35). A candidate, attenuated HSV-1/HSV-2 vaccine, entered phase I clinical studies in France within the last year.

Perhaps the most important infectious disease in the world, malaria, presents the most formidable challenge for vaccine development (36). The impact of malaria is difficult to estimate, but millions of people succumb to the disease each year. Although much is now known about the parasite and its biology, attempts to develop vaccines have been greatly complicated by the complex life cycle of the parasite, not only in the host, but also in the insect vector. The parasite expresses different antigenic determinants during different stages of its life cycle, and it has been difficult to determine which immune responses are protective in humans (37).

Early promise was generated by observations that immunity to the circumsporozoite (CS) was protective in man (38). This antigen has been cloned and studied not only as a purified protein, but also in subunits (39). Neither approach has proved effective in preventing infection, although early studies demonstrated that protection from experimental challenge could be obtained by exposure to irradiated circumsporozoites (38,40). Other studies have focused on the role of blood-stage antigens (41), and there is some evidence that vaccines containing a cocktail of blood-stage antigens may be protective (42). One innovative approach that has been proposed is to generate vaccines against the gametocyte antigens (43). It is thought that such vaccines would affect the ability of the parasite to reinfect the mosquito. This kind of vaccine would, in effect, control malaria indirectly by interrupting a critical step in the parasite's life cycle. Although there are many approaches to pursue in the development of a malaria vaccine, it is evident that effective malaria vaccines are still many years in the future. Many problems remain that will require a continuing commitment to basic research in malaria before solutions emerge.

Significant progress has also been made in the development of vaccines to prevent hepatitis A virus (HAV) (44), rotavirus (45), and varicella zoster (16), and in the development of polysaccharide-protein conjugate vaccines. Clinical trials to demonstrate the effectiveness of killed HAV vaccines are now being planned. Current candidate vaccines stimulate high levels of serum antibody. Since passive immunization is known to be effective in preventing HAV infections, it is highly likely that a vaccine that stimulates high levels of serum antibody will also be protective in this situation. A revolution in the design of polysaccharide vaccines is currently under way. The success of the *Haemophilus influenzae* PRP polysaccharide-protein conjugate vaccines has greatly stimulated research in this area (47-49). Candidate polysaccharide-protein conjugate vaccines for several important infections have been developed in the laboratory, including: pneumococcal polysaccharide conjugates, *Salmonella typhi* Vi polysaccharide-protein conjugates, and group B streptococcal (GBS) polysaccharide-protein conjugates (53). All these vaccines will require additional basic and clinical research before they are realities. However, the problems associated with the further development of the vaccines cited above are known, and significant progress will be made in the next decade on their development. Certainly one of the most important issues that requires resolution is the use of these vaccines in pregnant women. The utility of GBS polysaccharide vaccines will probably depend on the use of these vaccines in that population group, since the primary impact of GBS is in the immediate neonatal period.

CONCLUDING REMARKS

The future of vaccine research is a bright one. The scientific base and practical success of vaccination are unassailable. Basic research in infectious diseases, microbiology, and immunology will continue to open avenues of research and development that will directly and positively affect vaccine development efforts. It is important to note, however, that several areas need additional emphasis. One of these is the general area of mucosal immunity. This is critically important if effective vaccines to prevent STDs are to be developed. Emphasis also needs to be placed on research to combine antigens from different vaccines and to enhance the immunogenicity of vaccines. One potential approach to this problem is to use timed-release methodology to both enhance immunogenicity and reduce the number of doses required for protection. All these efforts will require a continued commitment to the integration of basic and clinical research activities, as well as a continuous requirement for field observations and epidemiology of vaccine-preventable diseases to identify new variants and to monitor efficacy and safety.

REFERENCES

1. Norrby E. Measles. In: Fields BN, ed. Virology. New York: Raven Press, 1985.
2. Fenner F, Henderson DA, Artia I, et al. Smallpox and Its Eradication. Geneva: World Health Organization, 1988.
3. Henderson DA. Smallpox and vaccinia. In: Plotkin SA, Mortimer EA, eds. Vaccines. Philadelphia: WB Saunders, 1988:8-30.
4. Hinman AR. Public health considerations. In: Plotkin SA, Mortimer EA, eds. Vaccines. Philadelphia: WB Saunders, 1988:587-603.
5. Paul JR. Epidemiology of Poliomyelitis. WHO Monograph Series No. 26. Geneva: World Health Organization, 1955:9-29.
6. Whooping Cough: Reports from the Committee on the Safety of Medicines and the Joint Committee on Vaccination and Immunisation. London: Department of Health and Social Security, Her Majesty's Stationery Office, 1981.
7. Griffith AH. Permanent brain damage and pertussis vaccination: is the end of the saga in sight? Vaccine 1989; 7:199-210.
8. Talwar GP, Hingorani V, Kumar S, Roy S, Banerjee A, Shahani SM, Krishna U, Dhall K, Sawhney H, Sharma NC, et al. Phase I clinical trials with three formulations of anti-human chorionic gonadotropin vaccine. Contraception 1990; 41(3):301-316.

9. Krugman S. Hepatitis B vaccine. In: Plotkin SA, Mortimer EA, eds. Vaccines. Philadelphia: WB Saunders, 1988:458-473.

10. Fedson DS. Pneumococcal vaccine. In: Plotkin SA, Mortimer EA, eds. Vaccines. Philadelphia: WB Saunders, 1988:271-299.

11. Yamanoto T, Yukota T. Electron microscopic study of *Vibrio cholerae* 01 adherence to the mucous coat and villus surface in the human small intestine. Infect Immunol 1988; 56:2753-2759.

12. Greenough WB III. *Vibrio cholerae.* In: Mandell GL, Douglas RG, Bennett JE, eds. Infectious Diseases and Their Etiologic Agents. Third Edition. New York: Churchill Livingstone, 1990:1636.

13. Britigan BE, Cohen MS, Sparling PF. Gonococcal infections: a model of molecular pathogenesis. N Engl J Med 1985; 312:1683-1694.

14. Centers for Disease Control. Recommendations of the Public Health Service Advisory Committee on Immunization Protection: Measles vaccines. MMWR 1967; 16:269-271.

15. Fine PE, Clarkson JA. Reflections on the efficacy of pertussis vaccines. Rev Infect Dis 1987; 9(5):866-883.

16. Gershon AA, Steinberg SP, Gelb L, Galasso G, et al., National Institute of Allergy and Infectious Diseases Varicella Vaccine Collaborative Study Group. Live attenuated varicella vaccine: Efficacy for children with leukemia in remission. JAMA 1984; 252:355-362.

17. Nathanson N, Langmuir AD. The Cutter incident: Poliomyelitis following formaldehyde-inactivated poliovirus vaccination in the United States during the spring of 1955. I. Background. Am J Hyg 1963; 78:16-28.

18. Morton DL, Foshag LJ, Nizze JA, et al. Active specific immunotherapy in malignant melanoma. Sem Surg Oncol 1989; 5(6):420-425.

19. Miller DL, Alderslade R, Ross EM. Whooping cough and whooping cough vaccine: the risks and benefits debate. Epidemiol Rev 1982; 4:1-24.

20. Kitch EW. American law and preventive vaccine programs. In: Plotkin SA, Mortimer EA, eds. Vaccines. Philadelphia: WB Saunders, 1988.

21. Noble GR, Bernier RH, Estes CE, et al. Acellular and whole-cell pertussis vaccines in Japan: Report of a visit by U.S. scientists. JAMA 1987; 257:1351-1356.

22. Nencioni L, Pizza MG, et al. Characterization of genetically inactivated pertussis toxin mutants: Candidates for a new vaccine against whooping cough. Sciences.

23. Isomura S. Clinical studies on efficacy and safety of acellular pertussis vaccine. Tokai J Exp Clin Med 1988; 13(suppl):39-43.

24. Ad Hoc Group for the Study of Pertussis Vaccines. Placebo-controlled trial of two acellular pertussis vaccines in Sweden—protective efficacy and adverse events. Lancet 1988; i:955-960; erratum appears in Lancet 1988; i:1238.

25. Kato T, Kaku H, Arimoto Y. Protection against pertussis by Takeda's acellular pertussis vaccine: household contact studies in Kawasaki City, Japan. Tokai J Exp Clin Med 1988; 13(suppl):35-38.

26. Koff WC, Hoth DF. Development and testing of AIDS vaccines. Sciences 1988; 241(4864):426-432.

27. Katzenstein DA, Sawyer LA, Quinnan GV. Human immunodeficiency virus. In: Plotkin SA, Mortimer EA, eds. Vaccines. Philadelphia: WB Saunders, 1988:558-567.

28. Brennan PW, Gregory TJ, Riddle L, et al. Protection of chimpanzees from infection by HIV-1 after vaccinations with recombinant glycoprotein gp120 but not gp160. Nature 345:622-625.

29. Clemens JD, Harris JR, Kay BA, Chakraborty J, Sack DA, Ansaruzzaman M, Rahman R, Stanton BF, Khan MU, Khan MR, et al. Oral cholera vaccines containing B-subunit-killed whole cells and killed whole cells only. II. Field evaluation of cross-protection against other members of the Vibrionaceae family. Vaccine 1989; 7(2):117-120.

30. Holmgren J, Clemens J, Sack DA, Svennerholm AM. New cholera vaccines. Vaccine 1989; 7(2):94-96.

31. Bagshawe A, Scott GC, Russell DA, Wigley SC, Merianos A, Berry G. BCG vaccination in leprosy: final results of the trial in Karimui, Papua New Guinea, 1963-79. Bull WHO 1989; 67(4):389-399.

32. Fine PE, Ponnighaus JM. Leprosy in Malawi. 2. Background, design and prospects of the Karonga Prevention Trial, a leprosy vaccine trial in northern Malawi. Trans R Soc Trop Med Hyg 1988; 82(6):810-817.

33. Deo MG, ICRC "anti-leprosy vaccine." Vaccine 1989; 7(2):92-93.

34. Mertz GJ, Ashley R, Burke RL, Benedetti J, Critchlow C, Jones CC, Corey L. Double-blind, placebo-controlled trial of a herpes simplex virus type 2 glycoprotein vaccine in persons at high risk for genital herpes infection. J Infect Dis 1990; 161(4):653-660.

35. Roizman B, Jenkins FJ. Genetic engineering of novel genomes of large DNA viruses. Science 1985; 229:1208-1214.

36. Zavala F, Tan JP, Hollingdale MR, Cochran AN, et al. Rationale for development of a synthetic vaccine against *Plasmodium falciparum* malaria. Science 1985; 228:1436-1440.

37. Cohen S. Review lecture—Immunity to malaria. Proc R Soc London Ser B 1979; 203:323-345.

38. Clyde DF, McCarthy VC, Miller RM, Woodward WF. Immunization of man against falciparum and vivax malaria by the use of attenuated sporozoites. Am J Trop Med Hyg 24:397-401.

39. Nardin EH, Nussenswig V, Nussenswig RS, Collins WE, Harimasuta KT, Tapachoisin P, Chomchant. Circumsporozoite proteins of human malaria parasites *Plasmodium falciparum* and *Plasmodium vivax*. J Exp Med 1982; 156:20-30.

40. Nussenswig V, Nussenswig RS. Sporozoite malaria vaccines. In: Englund PT, Sher A, eds. The Biology of Parasitism. New York: Alan R Liss, 1988: 183-199.

41. Andus RF. Antigens of *Plasmodium falciparum* and their potential as components of malaria vaccines. In: Englund PT, Sher A, eds. The Biology of Parasitism. New York: Alan R Liss, 1988:201-224.

42. Patarroyo ME, Romero P, Torres ML, Clavijo P, Moreno A, et al. Introduction of protective immunity against experimental infection with malaria using synthetic peptides. Nature 1987; 328:629-632.

43. Cater R. Immunity to seasonal stages of Malaria parasites in relation to malaria transmission. In: Englund PT, Sher A, eds. The Biology of Parasitism. New York: Alan R Liss, 1988:225-231.

44. Deinhardt F, Hillerman MR. Hepatitis A vaccine. In: Plotkin SA, Mortimer EA, eds. Vaccines. Philadelphia: WB Saunders, 1988:549-557.

45. Vesikari T, Rautanen T, Varis T, Beards GM, Kapikian AZ. Rhesus rotavirus candidate vaccine. Clinical trial in children vaccinated between 2 and 5 months of age. Am J Dis Child 1990; 144(3):285-289.

46. Bjune G, Nkleby H, Hareide B. Clinical trials of the new Norwegian vaccine against diseases caused by Meningococcus B. Tidsskr Nor Laegeforen 1990; 110(5):614-617.

47. Black SB, Shinefield HR. Efficacy of *Haemophilus influenzae* type b (b-CAPSA 1) polysaccharide vaccine in 87,541 children. Pedriat Res 1987; 21: 322a.

48. Osterholm MT, et al. Lack of protective efficacy and increased risk of disease within 7 days after vaccination associated with *Haemophilus influenzae* type b (Hib) polysaccharide (PS) vaccine use in Minnesota (MN). Abstract 318. Program and Abstracts of the 27th Interscience Conference on Antimicrobial Agents and Chemotherapy, New York, October 1-4, 1987.

49. Ward J, Brennemann G, Letson W, et al. Limited efficacy of a *Haemophilus influenzae* type b conjugate vaccine (PRP-D) in Alaskan native infants immunized at 2, 4, and 6 months of age. Lancet. In press.

50. Hoke CH, Nisalak A, Sangawhipa N, Jatanasen S, Laorakapongse T, Innis BL, Kotchasenee S, Gingrich JB, Latendresse J, Fukai K, et al. Protection against Japanese encephalitis by inactivated vaccines. N Engl J Med 1988; 319(10):608-614.

51. Aaby P, Jensen TG, Hansen HL, Kristiansen H, et al. Trial of high dose Edmonston-Zagreb measles vaccine in Guinea-Bissau: protective efficacy. Lancet 1988; ii:809-811.

52. Acharya IL, Lowe CU, Thapa R, Gurubacharya VL. Prevention of Typhoid fever in Nepal with the V. capsular polysaccharide of salmonella toxin. A preliminary report. N Engl J Med 1987; 317(18):1101-1104.

53. Baker CJ, Rench MA, Edwards MS, et al. Immunization of pregnant women with a polysaccharide vaccine. N Engl J Med 1988; 319:1180-1185.

8

The Development of an HIV Vaccine

Legal and Policy Aspects

Robert E. Stein
*Blicker Futterman & Stein
and Georgetown Law Center
Washington, D.C.*

INTRODUCTION

Society looks for magic bullets to combat disease. Vaccines are often thought of in this way, as the most effective disease combatant. Whether the disease is smallpox; childhood diseases including pertussis, diphtheria, and typhus; mumps, measles, and rubella; or polio, the belief has been that if there is a vaccine, and it is widely used, there is little to worry about.

In the United States, a number of legal and policy issues have had an influence on the development of vaccines. There are some reports that the legal system in the United States—in which litigation is often used by individuals seeking compensation and other damages for injuries suffered or believed to have been suffered as a result of taking or administering a vaccine—has inhibited the development and manufacture of vaccines. This chapter examines legal issues that have been raised in the development of

223

vaccines for a number of diseases and applies them to these issues as they may arise during the development of an HIV or AIDS vaccine. After dealing with liability concerns, I discuss informed consent and compensation for individuals injured as a result of taking a vaccine. Finally, suggestions for how these issues can be addressed in dealing with an AIDS vaccine are explored.

The need for an AIDS vaccine is clear. However, if HIV is to be stopped, a number of things are necessary. We must educate people so that they understand how HIV is transmitted, how it is not transmitted, and how they can protect themselves. We must have drugs to control, if not cure, HIV infection, and there is increasing progress toward achieving that goal. And we must have a vaccine that is safe and effective.

Recent progress indicates that there are candidate vaccines for which clinical trials make sense. Unlike other diseases, however, for which a vaccine is viewed as necessary, there are some who believe that for most individuals prevention against HIV infection through means other than vaccines may be more effective, and are certainly better developed. As June Osborn, Dean of the School of Public Health at the University of Michigan and Chair of the National Commission on AIDS, put it (1):

> The goal is not to make vaccines but to prevent HIV, and vaccines will play a role in that, and the question is how much of a role. . . . I hope we can do lots of other much more effective things so that we never reach the point where we need to be discussing the use of whatever vaccine as the primary or sole protective measure.

For this reason, in addition to the elusiveness of the AIDS vaccine itself, the difficulties encountered when developing any vaccine—questions relating to safety and effectiveness, the realities of time constraints and expense, and liability issues—are compounded for AIDS vaccine researchers by the problems that are unique to AIDS and HIV. These include dangers both known and unknown, difficulties related to insurability of HIV-infected individuals, societal misconception of AIDS and how it is transmitted, and whether volunteers in vaccine clinical trials pose an additional risk for transmission.

This chapter first sets forth the process of vaccine development, tracing its procedures and legal issues that have arisen. Next, it examines the obstacles encountered in the search for an HIV or AIDS vaccine, obstacles that are largely related to the nature of HIV. Finally, it concentrates on liability and other legal/policy issues presented by the development and use of an AIDS vaccine.

VACCINE DEVELOPMENT ISSUES

Experts in the field of drug and vaccine development estimate that it takes 10 years and $10 million to bring a vaccine to market in the United States today (2). The cost and time spent are the result of the research and testing required to develop a vaccine to the point that it can be used in human trials, and of the government's efforts to ensure safety to those who volunteer to test a vaccine.

According to the World Health Organization (WHO), the three clinical trial stages of development for an HIV vaccine—which in their scope and objectives would also apply to other vaccines that are under development—are as follows (3):

Phase I.   Phase I trials refer to the first introduction of the candidate vaccine preparation in the human population with the purpose of initial determination of its safety and biological effects including immunogenicity. This phase may include studies of dose and route of administration and usually involves less than 100 volunteers.

Persons included in this group should be healthy, HIV-seronegative individuals who have no recognized risk behavior for HIV infection. It is recommended that pregnant women be excluded from this group. All participants should be fully informed volunteers.

Phase II.   Phase II trials refer to the initial trials examining potential effectiveness in a limited number of volunteers (usually between 200 and 500 individuals). In the case of candidate vaccines, the principal focus of this phase is immunogenicity.

The target group should be made up of fully informed HIV-seronegative volunteers. It should include representation of all population groups that might be included in a phase III trial. Moreover, since in phase III trials HIV-positive individuals may receive vaccine, it may be appropriate to include a small group of such individuals in phase II trials. Participants must be prepared to avoid behaviors which place them at risk of acquiring HIV infection.

Phase III.   Phase III trials are intended to provide for a more complete assessment of safety and effectiveness in the prevention of disease, involving larger numbers of volunteers in a multi-centered, adequately controlled study.

These trials must satisfy the highest standards of scientific investigation. The study design should be appropriate to the vaccine and the study population. The ideal would be a controlled double blind, fully randomized trial. They should be performed in groups of individuals which represent all of the major routes of HIV infection (sexual, parental and mother to infant).

In the United States, in order to market a vaccine, researchers must gain the approval of the Food and Drug Administration (FDA) that the vaccine is safe for testing on humans (4). Next, researchers must find healthy volunteers who are willing to submit themselves to known and unknown risks.

FDA Requirements for Vaccine Testing

In order to gain approval from the FDA, all vaccines must be put through a three-phase clinical testing program similar to that suggested by WHO. However, before testing on human subjects can begin, the FDA requires that a new drug or vaccine be proven safe, and evidence of such safety includes studies on animals (5).

As with the WHO requirements referred to above, the final phase of testing, phase III, involves a far greater number of volunteers than used in earlier phases. The goal of phase III testing is to obtain statistics regarding a vaccine's safety and effectiveness. The volunteer group in phase III testing should represent all segments of the population who are at risk for the disease that the vaccine attempts to combat. While it is often this last stage that is focused on by groups eager to obtain a vaccine, according to the Pharmaceutical Manufacturers Association (PMA) the approval review time by the FDA is but a small portion of the total time required between the research phase and final approval (6).

In addition to following the regulations set forth by the FDA, researchers are faced with finding an adequate number of volunteers for testing. Beyond screening volunteers for risk behavior, researchers must honestly and fully inform potential volunteers of any risks that may be associated with the experimental vaccine.

Informed Consent

The statutory and common law of the United States requires that doctors obtain voluntary, full and informed consent from participants in medical research studies. There is some evidence that the concept of informed consent in the United States antedates the second World War (7). However, it was not until much more recently that rigor was introduced into the process. In recognition of the conflicting interests that research subjects and researchers often have, the requirement of informed consent is strictly applied in the vaccine-testing context. Factors contributing to the stringent application of the requirement are (8):

(1) Because the risks of experimentation are not known in advance, only the subject can decide whether to undergo them; (2) any argument for deferring to medical expertise is inappropriate in the research setting; (3) the research subject, who is unlikely to benefit directly from the research, cannot be presumed to consent to it; and (4) the research and the subject often have conflicting interests.

The formal practice of informed consent is relatively new in the United States. It was not until 1974 that the United States Congress created the National Commission for the Protection of Human Subjects of Biomedical and Behavioral Research, thereby establishing a formal system to review ethical aspects of proposed studies involving human subjects (9). Indeed, consider this description of the informed-consent process in the polio clinical trials in the 1950s (10):

Across the country, teachers explained the field trial in terms that a child of six or seven could understand. The vaccine had been developed by very careful scientists who wanted to help the children stay healthy. It was pink, and it came in little bottles. The shot would feel like a tiny prick, more than a mosquito bite, and would only hurt for a moment. No one would know how well it worked until next year. They were pioneers. Pioneers are special people who go first. They were lucky to be able to get vaccine.

In the eleven states that took part in the double-blind placebo trials, the explanations went further. Doctors needed to measure how well the vaccine worked, the children were told. To do that, they had to compare children who got vaccine to children who didn't. Nobody could know who got which, or the experiment would not come out right. Next year they would each find out what they had received. No one would know how well it worked until next year. They were all pioneers. Pioneers are special people who go first. They were all very lucky.

The FDA requirements for informed consent involve a statement that the study involves research, and its purposes, duration, and procedures; a description of reasonably foreseeable risks; a description of any benefits to the subject (which in the case of an experimental vaccine must be explained, as there may not be any benefit); a disclosure of appropriate alternative procedures; a statement about confidentiality; indication of whether compensation or medical treatments are available; and information about where to go for answers about rights (11). The subject must also be told that participation is voluntary and advised of the medical consequences of withdrawal. Moreover, the informed consent must be documented through the use of a written consent form approved by the Institutional Review Board and signed by the subject (12).

While informed consent is now routinely practiced in the United States, problems remain with experimental vaccine research. Although researchers are able to inform volunteers of known risks, they are faced with admitting to potential volunteers that even they do not know all the possible risks associated with the proposed vaccine. This may be especially true for AIDS vaccines, as the latency period for disease is many years. In addition, it is especially important that volunteers be counseled about the potential lack of benefit so they are aware that the risks of unsafe sexual or drug-use behavior are not diminished by taking an experimental candidate vaccine with unknown efficacy. Moreover, because of the findings of a number of courts that informed consent was not adequate in cases in which alternative treatment existed (13) or all known risks were not discussed (14), the informed consent process has evolved so that the avoidance of liability takes on as much importance as informing the patient or volunteer.

Liability for Injuries Caused by Vaccines: Established Doctrines and Emerging Trends

American law concerning drug manufacturer liability for injuries resulting from vaccines has evolved primarily from experience with the polio and DPT vaccines. It centers on two principal areas: a manufacturer's failure to warn vaccinees of possible dangers and defective or negligent vaccine design.

With regard to a failure on the part of a manufacturer to directly warn a vaccine recipient of dangers inherent in the vaccine, a strict liability standard has evolved over the last 25 years. In the case of *Davis v. Wyeth Laboratories* (15), a federal court of appeals held a polio vaccine manufacturer strictly liable for plaintiff's vaccine-related injuries when the manufacturer did not directly warn the plaintiff that use of its vaccine could lead to polio, as it did in plaintiff's case. This was extended by another federal appeals court in *Reyes v. Wyeth Laboratories* (16) to hold a polio vaccine manufacturer strictly liable for failure to directly warn a vaccinee when the vaccine's package insert warned hospital staff members of potential dangers and the staff did not pass these warnings on to the plaintiff, who contracted polio from the vaccine. The strict liability standard for failure to warn has been cited as the reason for both a reduction in the number of manufacturers of DPT vaccine and a dramatic increase in the price of that vaccine (17).

In a challenge to these cases, there are signs of a trend to not impose strict liability in vaccine cases in which the manufacturer did not directly warn the vaccinee, on the grounds that a vaccine is "unavoidably unsafe." Under this liability defense theory, shaped by tort and contract law, urgent societal need for a product is weighed against the product's inherent dangers, both known and unknown. The American Law Institute, a private body in the United States that restates the law in different areas, and whose work is given great weight by the courts, examined the issue of "unavoidably unsafe" products in its Restatement (second) of Torts. Under Comment k to §402A of the Restatement ("Comment k"), which sets forth the doctrine, a plaintiff bringing suit after a vaccine injury will probably prevail if the product is improperly prepared, or inadequate instructions or warnings as to known adverse effects were given (18).

There is, however, criticism of the way in which state legislatures determine a product to be "unavoidably unsafe." In order to determine whether a product is "unavoidably unsafe," a California appeals court in *Kearl v. Lederle Laboratories* (19) formulated this three-part test (20):

1. Whether, when distributed, the product was intended to confer an exceptionally important benefit that made its availability highly desirable
2. Whether the then-existing risk posed by the product was both "substantial" and "unavoidable"
3. Whether the interest in availability (again measured as of the time of distribution) outweighs the interest in promoting enhanced accountability through strict liability design-defect review

In an effort to encourage development of an AIDS vaccine, the State of California enacted a statute that incorporates these criteria to determine whether a product is "unavoidably unsafe," in the hope of safeguarding AIDS vaccine manufacturers from a burdensome liability (21).

Another challenge to the strict liability norm that manufacturers have a duty to warn vaccinees of dangers inherent in the vaccine is found in the "learned intermediary" doctrine, which contends that a direct manufacturer's warning to the patient is unnecessary when a physician prescribes a drug because the prescription entails an assessment of medical risks based on the physician's knowledge of his or her patient's needs and susceptibilities, and is therefore a medical choice (22). Under this doctrine, directly contrary to the *Reyes* decision, the relevant issue is whether the drug manufacturer adequately warned the *physician* of the drug's risks (23). Critics of the "learned intermediary" doctrine argue that it incorrectly presumes that the physician can be relied on to give the appropriate risk information to a patient, when in fact little information is provided with prescription drugs or vaccines and many patients report that they were never informed of risks by their physicians (24).

Applying both the "unavoidably unsafe" and the "learned intermediary" doctrine, a state court in *Johnson v. American Cyanamid* (25) found that a polio vaccine was "unavoidably unsafe," and in order to impose liability on its manufacturer for failure to warn, a plaintiff would have to prove negligence by the manufacturer. The court found that the manufacturer had given adequate warnings to the intermediary physician, sufficient to preclude manufacturer liability.

Although in most cases the central issue is whether adequate warning of attendant risks have been provided to the right party, persons injured by vaccines thought to be safe have sought relief alleging a defective design or negligent manufacturing.

Under the negligent manufacturing theory, when a manufacturer sells a vaccine in a condition other than that specified under FDA approval, and the difference causes an adverse reaction, that product was considered to have been negligently manufactured. While reported decisions in which this theory of liability is used are rare, in one case involving a polio vaccine the court implied to the finding of negligent manufacturing (26):

> If the vaccine is produced as it should be it must be free of virulent particles, that is, all of the particles should be attenuated or nonvirulent . . . if the vaccine did cause plaintiff's illnesses, the inference is warranted that the vaccine did contain virulent particles, and, therefore, that it was defective.

The design defect theory, as rare in its litigation appearance as the negligent manufacture theory, hinges on the intentional inclusion of an inappropriate or inadequately tested component in a vaccine as approved by the FDA. This theory has been successful when an inappropriate and inadequately tested preservative caused the release of an infectious endotoxin into the vaccine, which ultimately led to brain damage (27).

Toner v. Lederle Laboratories (28) added a twist to the defective design theory of liability, when a vaccine manufacturer was effectively held liable for designing the wrong vaccine. A pertussis vaccine manufacturer, who marketed the only pertussis vaccine licensed by the FDA, was held liable for negligent design when a differently designed vaccine could have been developed. Although such a vaccine had been denied approval by the FDA, the court suggested that more effort on the manufacturer's part might have led to approval.

One question that remains to be answered is whether a manufacturer will be held liable under a theory of defective design when an unforeseeable adverse effect ultimately causes its risks to outweigh its benefits.

Concern about liability has been cited by pharmaceutical companies among their reasons for leaving the vaccine market. It was in an effort to stop this market flight, and to ensure compensation for the injured, that the National Childhood Vaccine Injury Act (NCVIA) of 1986 (29), discussed below, was introduced and approved by Congress in 1986.

SPECIAL ISSUES RAISED BY AIDS

While development of a safe and effective vaccine to prevent HIV infection is of fundamental importance in the battle to halt the spread of AIDS, general difficulties are posed by HIV that have generated obstacles to the successful development of a vaccine. Some companies have maintained that liability concerns have limited their interest in a vaccine, although proof of this is hard to demonstrate (30).

Because of the nature of the AIDS epidemic—the nature of the virus itself, and the fact that HIV-infected individuals are often discriminated against within our society—the quest for a vaccine has faced obstacles which other vaccine searches have not. Several medical, legal, and ethical questions are raised with regard to an AIDS vaccine that are not posed with other vaccines.

There have been a number of vaccine candidates for which clinical trials have begun. For example, on November 20, 1990, the National Institute of Allergy and Infectious Diseases (NIAID) announced that it had received approval from the FDA to begin human clinical trials of a new candidate AIDS vaccine, which will undergo clinical testing in NIAID's network of five AIDS Vaccine Evaluation Units (AVEUs) (31). In phase I testing, by random assignment, 20 volunteers will receive the real vaccine and 10 will receive a placebo, with neither the volunteers nor the study physicians knowing who is receiving which vaccine (32). The use of informed consent mechanisms, as noted above, is extensive.

Medical Issues Presented by AIDS Vaccine Testing

The HIV virus poses obstacles to the development of a successful vaccine, as the virus itself is elusive: It can lie dormant for years, hiding in cells and mutating into strains that are not affected by the vaccine being tested. Because AIDS is presumed fatal in every case, a vaccine must be without risk of causing HIV infection, which for many researchers rules out vaccines made using a purified form of the live virus (33). As HIV is a new and exceedingly complex virus, there is the possibility that established vaccine approaches will require modification (34). There are now several strains of HIV, and although a vaccine may be successful against one strain of the virus, the same virus might self-mutate into a strain that the same vaccine cannot combat. This forces researchers to search for a vaccine that will work against both known and unknown HIV strains.

Moreover, no vaccine is 100% effective. Public health officials have asked how effective a vaccine will have to be to replace other known means of prevention of transmission, including safer sex practices and cleaning, or not sharing, needles. In fact, it is argued, that except where a society has a very high incidence, vaccines will only have a limited use (35).

The three-phase FDA trial process poses a problem to AIDS vaccine research. Specifically, phase III is problematic: With the level of HIV infection in the United States relatively low at present, it is possible that efficacy trials will require the participation of thousands of people and extend over several years (36). One proposed way to reduce the trial size and duration is to perform phase II and phase III trials in countries where the HIV infection rate is higher than in the United States (37). If this is done—and it is believed that trials will have to take place in Africa or other developing countries in order to obtain an indication of significant reductions in infection through the vaccine (38)—new legal and ethical issues will arise. Do the laws of potential countries for trials formulate or pose obstacles to those trials? How should informed consent be treated in countries with diverse backgrounds? How will counseling be addressed to ensure that volunteers also understand behavioral changes that will assist in risk reduction?

In addition, it is considered to be nearly impossible to forecast the scope of the risks associated with the development and marketing of an AIDS vaccine, and it is generally assumed that the risks associated with an AIDS vaccine may be less predictable and potentially more serious than the risks associated with other vaccines (39). If the latency period for injuries from an AIDS vaccine extends for years, in the same manner as the latency period of AIDS itself, researchers will not know the full spectrum of vaccine-related risks for perhaps more than a decade (40).

Another medical dilemma posed in the search for an AIDS vaccine is the absence of an animal model for the disease. Relatively few animals can be infected with the HIV virus and, of those that can, none provide an exact match to the human system with regard to the symptoms generated by HIV (41). Therefore, researchers cannot rely, as they have in the past with other vaccines, on animals to definitely predict whether a particular immunogen can eradicate HIV in humans. Following initial in vitro experimentation, man must serve as his own experimental animal for an AIDS vaccine (42). Is it courageous or foolhardy to allow uninfected individuals to be treated with experimental vaccines whose safety has not yet been ascertained without a better model?

While the medical obstacles involved in the researching and testing of AIDS vaccines are arduous, there are nonmedical obstacles to research that are equally compelling. Representative of such obstacles are the legal and ethical problems associated with mandatory reporting requirements, informed consent, and human-subject testing.

Legal and Ethical Issues: Reporting Requirements, Informed Consent, and Human-Subject Experimentation

An accurate database chronicling the number of HIV-infected individuals is of paramount importance in the fight against AIDS. Yet there is disagreement as to whether the names of HIV infected individuals should be reported as well as their HIV-positive status: Notions of privacy and of individual liberty sound alarms for some that, if in the wrong hands, the knowledge that a person is HIV-positive can do a great deal of personal and professional damage (43). This has implications for individuals who volunteer for clinical trials for an AIDS vaccine.

A number of states have enacted reporting requirements whereby the names of HIV-positive individuals are to be reported to state public health authorities (44). One state with mandatory reporting has an exception for individuals participating in research projects whereby the fact of positivity must be reported by the research center that tests the individual, but it can be done anonymously. The state has concluded that a person applying to volunteer in an HIV clinical trial program who tests positive during the initial screening will be considered a participant in a research program, so that his or her names does not have to be supplied to public authorities. Reporting requirements may well serve as an obstacle in the search for an effective vaccine against AIDS, as some potential volunteers will avoid the trials in order to avoid the stigma associated with revealing to the state their HIV-positive status after vaccination. This will be increasingly important in phase II and III trials in which seropositive volunteers will be sought.

Another obstacle to volunteer participation is posed by the vaccine trial method itself. For phase I and early phase II trials, volunteers must be HIV-free, and not be at high risk of contacting the disease. All must be willing to have blood drawn. Volunteers go through an extensive interview and informed-consent process, with probative questions regarding their sexual history, sexual practices, and history of drug use.

Because persons immunized with an AIDS vaccine will test positive for HIV, they may be subjected to social discrimination, encountering resistance if they try to donate blood, enter a foreign country, or join the military or foreign service (45). Some potential volunteers have been reported to have experienced other forms of discrimination, for example, told they will be fired from their jobs if they participate in a vaccine trial, or that they will not be covered by their insurance for complications that may result from their trial participation (46).

If, as indicated above, clinical trials are conducted outside the United States, there are applicable U.S. regulations on the protection of human research subjects. While in some countries, it may be difficult to organize an institutional review board to oversee the trials, what is being sought is an indication that each subject is provided information about: the purpose of the study; reasonable, foreseeable risks; any benefits to the subject; appropriate alternative procedures; confidentiality of records; compensation, if any, of medical treatment information; and where to go for further information. Each subject should also understand that participation is voluntary (47). It remains to be seen how difficult it will be to reach the substance of these standards for trials conducted outside the United States.

LIABILITY ISSUES

There are several possibilities for harm with an AIDS vaccine that point to the issue of liability. Every volunteer is confronted with the risk of injury during trials or marketing: The risk of receiving a ''bad batch'' of the vaccine, the risk of negligence or fraud on the part of the researcher, the possibility that the subject will not be fully informed of the risks involved with the vaccine, or that the vaccine will not be as effective as thought. Is the volunteer entitled to compensation and, if so, who will compensate the volunteer for the physical and psychological injuries that may result from the vaccine?

The effects, both positive and negative, of an AIDS vaccine are at this point unknown. But if something goes awry, who will pay? What should be compensated—medical expenses, lost wages, pain and suffering? And *who* should pay? The individual, adequately apprised of the risks involved? The government, who allowed research to move forward? Drug companies, individually or collectively? Insurance carriers, through normal health and life coverage? Answers to these questions can assist in increasing willingness to participate of potential volunteers.

Who Will Compensate?

Any approach to compensation needs to be fair and equitable to both those who are asked to pay and those who are injured by a vaccine.

Litigation has been one of the principal means by which vaccine liability disputes have been resolved. In the area of HIV-related vaccine disputes, as with others, there are reasons that, for many cases, litigation may not be the most appropriate mechanism. It takes time, the transactional costs are high, and the results are uncertain. If there is a perceived risk of injury, no matter how small, the lack of a compensation system could dissuade individuals from participating in trials. This may not be as evident during early phase I trials, in which many volunteers have expressed humanitarian concern as a motivation for participation, but may well be more so during the phase II and III trials, in which there is a need to reach a broader audience.

While in other areas it may have been possible to obtain insurance to cover the risk of injuries, both during clinical trials and afterward, insurance specifically to cover vaccine injuries during the clinical trial phase of an AIDS vaccine has, to now, been extremely difficult to obtain. The liability system in the United States is considered too open-ended to be able to predict possible liability exposure. In contrast to vaccines with a history of use, with which there is an understanding of the kinds of injuries that might result, there is at present no such understanding with an AIDS vaccine.

In some countries, existing law may provide a somewhat smaller degree of protection to vaccine recipients than may be considered appropriate according to ethical principles—thus, it may be desirable to consider enacting new law. The World Health Organization Expert Group consultation meeting in 1989 urged the adoption of guidelines to provide compensation for injured clinical-trial participants when the causal link is established between the trial and the injury. Elements of compensation should include medical and associated expenses and reimbursement for lost wages (48). These guidelines had earlier been urged by the Council for International Organizations of Medical Sciences but had not been implemented.

The specific form that a compensation system will take and the source of funds for paying that compensation remain to be worked out. Both federal legislative enactments in the related area of childhood vaccines and private initiatives in the AIDS vaccine area have resulted in approaches that are shaping the debate as to how individuals injured during clinical trials or after a vaccine is marketed should be compensated. Two options for compensation systems are 1) an exclusive compensation system and 2) a non-exclusive compensation system with modifications taken from tort law.

How effective would compensation schemes be in dealing with these kinds of cases? The National Childhood Vaccine Act provides an example to be closely examined to determine its applicability to cases involving injury from an HIV vaccine. Approved by Congress in 1986, the Act was not funded until later. Consequently, experience is only now developing with the claims under the Act. The Act initially provides an administrative remedy, with an appeal available to a tort action, in which state law would apply (49). The Act provides for compensation for medical expenses over $1000, loss of earnings, and up to $250,000 in the event of death caused by vaccination for childhood disease.

As there is a great deal of experience with the injuries from childhood vaccines, the legislation includes a table of injuries and compensation for them (50). The number of cases filed under the legislation has been higher than expected and the time extended for early filings (51). In the first annual report of the Special Masters (52), judgment was entered in 57 of the 92 cases completed. The Court of Claims entered judgments averaging about $480,000. It took about 10 months for a case to be heard by both a master and a judge. No petitioner refused the award to pursue a tort case, although four cases were appealed. It is not clear whether these cases will be reflective of the second or third hundred that will follow. As above, the number of cases filed has been higher than expected and the time extended for early filings (53).

An exclusive system would provide compensation for certain, well-defined losses (54), in addition to attorneys' fees, with an agreed-upon cap on recovery for pain and suffering. Payments would be made from a trust fund, administered by an appropriate agency, and decisions regarding disbursement of funds would be made by an independent decision-maker. By subrogating the trust fund to the rights of a person injured as a result of participating in an AIDS vaccine trial, current high standards of behavior by vaccine manufacturers and administrators could be maintained. Under this exclusive approach, a claimant would not be required to show fault on the part of the administrators or manufacturers of the vaccine, but would have to show causation—that the vaccine actually caused the injury.

Under a nonexclusive compensation with modified tort law scheme, an injured volunteer would make an irrevocable decision at the outset of the compensation process to either enter the compensation program or pursue a claim through the tort system. Through sufficient incentives to encourage most injured parties to pursue the compensation option rather than the modified tort option, parties would be assured of reasonable and efficient awards, while the tort approach could be reserved for cases strong enough to withstand the tougher tort system (55).

If a national compensation system for AIDS vaccine clinical-trial volunteers is established, the mechanism for financing any approach to compensation must be designed to provide the necessary funds both for current claims and to sustain the system into the future (56). Two approaches to be considered for a trust fund are initial funding provided by levying an excise tax on each HIV dose, or a loan or grant of federal seed money, which could be accumulated until needed.

A volunteer injured as a result of participation in a trial with a vaccine candidate should be compensated for losses suffered. Which losses, and how much compensation, for how long, are other questions.

A group under the auspices of the Keystone Center in Colorado, representing virtually all interested parties, recently issued a report on AIDS vaccine liability. One initial question posed by the group was "Are HIV vaccines similar to or different from those for other diseases?" In comparing a potential AIDS vaccine and the risks present in its development with other vaccines, the report states that "an AIDS vaccine can be expected to present similar, if not worse liability problems" (57).

But the group proceeded, because of a shared belief that it was worthwhile to address the liability issues now, *before* a crisis occurs, and to develop legal frameworks to govern AIDS vaccine-related injuries that could form the basis of further discussion and possible legislative action.

The report divided its analysis into two areas, focusing on the clinical trial stage and the eventual marketing of an AIDS vaccine. It recognized the importance of informed consent for both areas. In the past, most writing and virtually all litigation had focused on marketed vaccines. The Keystone group was in the vanguard in its consideration of clinical issues involved with an AIDS vaccine.

The system proposed would not cover conversion to HIV positivity resulting from other activities (e.g., it would not guarantee the effectiveness of the vaccine), and the group recognized that that issue must be brought out during the informed-consent process. Also, it was made clear to those participating that with the vaccines currently under clinical trial—which are predominantly envelope vaccines with genetically engineered material—there is no danger of contacting AIDS from the vaccine itself.

For marketed vaccines, the Keystone group recognized that the issues were different from those of the clinical-trial phase. Among the antecedents looked to was state legislation in California that provides for compensation for those injured by experimental vaccines, with a $250,000 cap. The state also undertook to purchase at least a half million doses of vaccine at $20 a dose. Not surprisingly, while the Keystone group could agree on basis principles to govern any system, they put forward two options—the first, an exclusive compensation system, called for compensation for unreimbursable medical costs, lost earnings, and pain and suffering. Payment would come from a trust fund.

The second option called for a nonexclusive compensation system with claimants using either the tort system or the compensation scheme. It would require an election. It was expected that people who chose the tougher standard of the tort system would be those with stronger cases.

The report of the Keystone Center builds on the examples in the National Childhood Vaccine Act to structure a specific set of approaches, although not always an agreed-upon one, to deal with an injury from an HIV vaccine.

As recently pointed out in the third report of the National AIDS Commission, there is a need to accelerate research and development on drugs and vaccines (58). There is a corresponding need to ensure that companies, including small companies without a large backup of resources, are not deterred from working toward a vaccine principally because of liability concerns.

In addition, there is a need to ensure that individuals participating in clinical trials are assured that their participation in those trials will not, if injury results, leave them without appropriate compensation for medical and economic losses. And there is a need to ensure that companies participating in vaccine trials, as well as later in the manufacture of a vaccine, are kept to a high standard, but that if injuries result, as seems to be inevitable, compensation will be provided.

Therefore, the schemes proposed by the Keystone report recognize that liability and compensation concerns are at least a significant factor in the development of vaccines. The report also recognizes that there is an inherent public benefit in encouraging the development of safe and effective vaccines and that, therefore, there is a role for compensation for individuals who are injured by a vaccine, whether at the clinical-trial stage or at the manufacturing stage.

As the report's section on funding options concludes, there are still too many uncertainties concerning expected side effects and how often they will occur, as well as the appropriate cap for maximum recovery, to draw up a final equation. It provides the most developed proposal to date to address this difficult problem.

Another possible compensation scheme is federal legislation to establish a compensation program to cover injuries incurred in both clinical trials and market use of an AIDS vaccine. There are two models for such legislation. One, enacted by the California legislature (59), provides that a manufacturer of an FDA-approved AIDS vaccine shall not be liable in strict product liability for any damages caused by a design or warning defect. It also includes an AIDS Vaccine Victims Compensation Fund to provide assistance to those injured by vaccination with an FDA-approved AIDS vaccine; the fund, however, is not available for injuries sustained during clinical trials (60). The second is the National Childhood Vaccine Act, discussed above, but it too is directed toward approved vaccines.

Insurability of Vaccine Trial Volunteers

While issues relating to liability continue to attract the most attention, a number of other legal issues have already surfaced that can influence the willingness of a volunteer to participate in vaccine trials. One of these concerns is eligibility for health and life insurance. Two issues that have been raised by volunteers are: the eligibility for insurance itself and reimbursement for medically necessary and appropriate treatment for complications that may result from participation in the trial.

The experience of the NIH as the administrator of trials has resulted in procedures to deal with these issues. The NIH provides all its volunteers with a tamper-proof identification card that includes a photograph.

NIAID maintains a computer registry of volunteers. Through a toll-free telephone number, verification of a volunteer's participation may be obtained with his concurrence. With this as background, the Institute has contacted the principal health insurance associations in the country—the Health Insurance Association of America (commercial insurers), the American Council of Life Insurance (life insurance commercial carriers), Blue Cross/Blue Shield of America (the association of the 78 regional Blue Cross and Blue Shield plans), and the Group Health Association of America (GHAA) (the trade association for Health Maintenance Organizations). Each of these groups has sent its members a letter from the NIH vaccine branch seeking concurrence that vaccine-trial volunteers who test positive under the ELISA and Western blot tests, as long as they have appropriate documentation, will not be discriminated against when only vaccine-induced antibodies are present in the Western blot. This is especially important, as a CDC-approved method of interpreting a positive Western blot test can include antibodies induced by a vaccine (61).

The second insurance issue that has been raised by volunteers is whether reimbursement will be provided for medically necessary and appropriate treatment for complications that may result from participation in the trial. here too, the Vaccine Research and Development branch sought confirmation of insurance companies' coverage for this care provided by a volunteer's own physician for a fee charged to the volunteer, and not for care provided by the clinical trial staff itself.

Given the large number of health-care providers in the country, it was felt that this mailing was the most effective way to apprise individual companies and other health-care providers of the scope and plans for the vaccine development program.

Thus far, there have been well over one hundred responses. There has been virtual unanimity with respect to the first question—that an individual participating in a trial will not be discriminated against because of HIV tests in which only vaccine-induced antibodies are present. Of the responding companies from Blue Cross/Blue Shield, the large majority have indicated that they will reimburse for the necessary and appropriate treatment for vaccine-related complications, as did those participants from GHAA.

Among the commercial carriers, there was widespread support for reimbursement when the complications were unexpected. For those that were expected and anticipated, while these companies normally do not cover those costs, they have indicated that they would review claims on a case-by-case basis.

This survey and the resulting responses were important because of the concerns of volunteers, some of whom had been told by their employers that they would lose their insurance as well as some who were concerned about possibly losing their jobs if they participated in a trial.

This issue raised a related concern, that of interpretation by CDC of the Western blot test, which, given the vaccines currently in use, could result in a test considered positive even though the antibodies are not virus-induced but vaccine-induced. NIH is seeking a clarification of this problem that will seek to advise readers of the MMWR of possible concerns with reading the test. For these reasons, the documentation provided to volunteers as part of the informed-consent process is very important.

Another issue that should be considered is that of testing for other insurance purposes. There may be a number of reasons for a volunteer at some point after he or she has participated in a clinical trial to take a Western blot test. If, as noted above, a reading is positive, that individual may not be eligible for certain jobs (foreign service or the military), may be denied entry into certain countries for travel, study, or work, or may even, if convicted of a federal crime in a jurisdiction where an HIV test is required for all inmates in state or federal penitentiaries, be put into an HIV-positive wing of the prison facility, should that exist. For this reason, it is important that the identification card be used and that NIH maintain the ability to confirm an individual's participation in a trial long into the future.

When trials are internationalized, there will be a number of additional legal issues to be resolved. For instance, Do the laws or administrative procedures of the host country or of the United States, such as those dealing with informed consent, operate as inhibitors?

As with the liability and compensation concerns, there are no simple answers to these questions. What remains clear is that legal issues designed to protect individuals may also hinder the search for volunteers and the willingness of companies to go forward. Attempting to anticipate these issues and seeking ways to deal with them may provide the best answers to ensuring that legal issues do not prove an impediment to the conduct of well-constructed, safe trials and the development of a safe, effective, and widely distributed vaccine.

CONCLUSION

It is not too early for interested groups, including Congress, to begin to consider what approaches will help society strike the balance required in the liability area. There is a need to ensure that companies large and small are not deterred from developing a vaccine because of liability concerns. There is a need to assure individuals participating in clinical trials that their participation will not, if injury results, leave them exposed, without appropriate coverage for medical and economic losses—if this is their perception, recruiting volunteers will be even more difficult than it is currently. And with these issues, the role of a safe and effective vaccine for AIDS in the context of an overall HIV-prevention strategy, both within the United States and globally, must be considered.

It is believed that there is an inherent public benefit in encouraging the development of safe and effective vaccines and, as the possibility of developing a safe and effective AIDS vaccine becomes more realistic, issues that have been put to the side need to be answered so that they will not hinder progress toward a safe and effective vaccine. In the quest for a vaccine, researchers must heed the necessary safety precautions that have been imposed by the FDA. The scientific community must also confront the legal, medical, and ethical dilemmas that are not present in the quest for other vaccines, as the true success and use of an AIDS vaccine as part of an HIV-prevention strategy is dependent on their resolution.

ACKNOWLEDGMENT

I would like to thank Claudia Callaway, J.D., Georgetown University, 1991, for her assistance in the preparation of this chapter.

REFERENCES

1. From a meeting of the Institute of Medicine Roundtable, September 10, 1990. Reprinted in AIDS Reference Guide Sec 1322 at 1 and 17.
2. Groves M. AIDS vaccine: Do we know where we are going? Pharm Tech July 1988:16.
3. World Health Organization. Statement from the Consultation on Criteria for International Testing of Candidate HIV Vaccines. Geneva, February 27-March 2, 1989. GPA/INF/89.8.
4. 23 CFR 312.23(a)(8) (1987).
5. *Ibid.*
6. Pharmaceutical Manufacturers Association. AIDS Products in Development. Winter 1990:7.
7. Faden R, Beauchamp T. A History of Informed Consent. New York: Oxford University Press, 1986:56.

8. Delgado R, Laskovac H. Informed consent in human experimentation: Bridging the gap between ethical thought and current practice. UCLA Law Rev 1986; 34:67.
9. Meulemans C. The Development of an AIDS Vaccine: Legal and Ethical Dilemma. Paper for Stein RE, Georgetown University Law Center, 1989:11.
10. Smith J. Patenting the Sun. New York: Knopf, 1990.
11. 45 CFR § 46.116.
12. *Id.* at § 46.117(a).
13. *See generally, Blanton v. U.S.,* 428 F.Supp. 360 (D.C. 1977) (in absence of plaintiff's consent, U.S. liable for administering experimental drug of unknown effectiveness when drug of known effectiveness and proven reliability was available).
14. *See generally, Wooderson v. Ortho Pharmaceutical Corp.,* 235 Kan. 387, 681 P.2d 1038, *cert. denied,* 105 S.Ct. 365 (1984) (even where manufacturer's warning referred to reaction equally or more serious and equally or more common, failure to mention specific reaction suffered by plaintiff is basis for liability); *see also, Davis v. Wyeth Laboratories,* 399 F.2d 121 (9th Cir. 1968) (even where risk of injury from use of drug is one in a million such risk must be disclosed by manufacturer).
15. 399 F.2d 121 (9th Cir. 1968).
16. 498 F.2d 1264 (5th Cir. 1974).
17. McKenna R. The impact of product liability in development of a vaccine against the AIDS virus. U Chicago Law Rev 1988; 55:943-964, at 955. During the 1960s, eight companies manufactured DPT vaccine and sold it for 11¢ a dose; by 1986, only one company manufactured the vaccine and sold it for $11 a dose.
18. American Law Institute Restatement 2nd Torts § 402A Comment K (1988).
19. 172 Cal.App.3d 812, 218 Cal.Rptr. 453 (Cal. App. 1st Dist. 1985).
20. *Id.* at 464.
21. Cal. Health & Safety Code chap. 1.14 (West Supp. 1988).
22. *Davis v. Wyeth Laboratories, supra,* note 15, at 130. "Learned intermediary" made its legal debut in *Sterling Drug, Inc. v. Cornish,* 370 F.2d 82, 85 (1966).
23. McKenna R, *supra*, note 17, at 959.
24. Gilhooley M. Learned Intermediaries, Prescription Drugs, and Patient Information, 1986.
25. 716 P.2d 1318 (Kan. 1986).
26. *Grinnell v. Charles Pfizer & Co.,* 274 Cal.App.2d 424, 79 Cal.Rptr. 369, 374 (Dist. Ct. App. 1969).
27. *Tinnerhold v. Parke Davis & Co.,* 285 F.Supp. 432 (S.D.N.Y. 1968).
28. 732 P.2d 297 (Id. 1987).
29. 42 U.S.C.A. §3000aa *et seq.* (1990).
30. The Keystone Center. Keystone AIDS Vaccine Liability Project Final Report (hereinafter Keystone Report), 1990:1.

31. News release, Health and Human Services, October 20, 1990:1.

32. *Id.* at 2.

33. Mariner W, Gallo C. Such vaccines carry a small risk of containing a live virus. Getting to Market: The Scientific and Legal Climate for Developing an AIDS Vaccine. Law, Med. and Health Care 1987; 15:1-2 at 17.

34. Keystone Report, *supra*, note 30, at 2.

35. Osborn, who stated: Institute of Medicine Roundtable, *supra*, note 1, What will a vaccine be perceived as a license to do, and how are we going to fix that.

36. Fauci A, Fischinger P. The development of an AIDS vaccine: Progress and promise. Public Health Reports 1988; 103:230, 234.

37. *Id.* at 235. However, variations in strains of HIV, discussed *supra*, may present additional obstacles to such trials.

38. National Institutes of Health. The AIDS Research Program of the NIH, 1991:59.

39. Keystone Report, *supra*, note 30, at 2.

40. Fauci A, Fischinger P. The mean incubation period for AIDS in adults is up to 8-10 years between initial infection with HIV and the development of clinical AIDS, *supra*, note 36, at 234.

41. Keystone Report, *supra*, note 30, at 2.

42. Groves M, *supra*, note 2, at 18.

43. *See e.g., Woods v. White,* 689 F.Supp. 874 (W.D. Wis. 1988) (constitutional right to privacy extends to fact that prison inmate has AIDS, and inmate retains the right during incarceration); *Doe v. Borough of Barrington*, No. 88-2642 (Dist.N.J. 1990) (police officers who told plaintiff's neighbors that plaintiff was infected with HIV violated plaintiff's constitutional right to privacy).

44. Gostin LO. All states require reporting of AIDS, as defined by the CDC, to the public health department; Arizona, Colorado, Florida, Georgia, Idaho, Indiana, Iowa, Kansas, Kentucky, Michigan, Minnesota, Mississippi, Missouri, Montana, Oklahoma, Rhode Island, South Carolina, Texas, Utah, Virginia, Wisconsin and Wyoming require the reporting of HIV-positive test results. Public Health Strategies for Confronting AIDS—Legislative and Regulatory Policy in the United States. JAMA 1989; 261(11):1626.

45. Fauci A, Fischinger P, *supra*, note 36, at 234.

46. Discussions of author with principal investigators, AIDS Vaccine Evaluation Groups.

47. 21 CFR 50 (1988).

48. WHO Expert Report, *supra*, note 3, at para. 2.3(b).

49. The Keystone Report, *supra*, note 30, borrows from the NCVA scheme in developing a policy to deal with injury from an HIV vaccine.

50. The AIDS Research Program of the NIH, *supra*, note 38, at p. 59 (1991).

51. Annual Report of the NCVA 1990, January 1991.

52. Office of the Special Masters, Annual Report, November 19, 1988-January 31, 1990.

53. Annual Report of the NCVA 1990, *supra*, note 51.
54. *E.g.*, unreimbursable medical and related expenses, lost earnings, pain and suffering.
55. Fauci A, Fischinger P, *supra*, note 36, at 19.
56. *Id.* at 18.
57. Keystone Report, *supra*, note 30, at 2.
58. The AIDS Research Program of the NIH, *supra*, note 38, at p. 58 (1991).
59. Cal. Health & Safety Code chap. 1.14, *supra*, note 21.
60. Mariner W, Gallo R, *supra*, note 33, at 24.
61. Morbidity and Mortality Weekly Report 1989; 38(S-7 1-6):3.

Index

About the Editors

Wayne C. Koff is Chief of the Vaccine Research and Development Branch, Division of AIDS, National Institute of Allergy and Infectious Diseases, National Institutes of Health, Bethesda, Maryland. The author or coauthor of numerous journal articles on vaccine development, he is a member of the American Association for the Advancement of Science, American Society for Microbiology, American Association of Immunologists, and Society for Clinical Trials. Dr. Koff received the B.A. degree (1974) in biology from Washington University, St. Louis, Missouri, and the Ph.D. degree (1979) in microbiology and immunology from the Baylor College of Medicine, Houston, Texas.

Howard R. Six is Vice President, Research and Development, Connaught Laboratories Inc., Swiftwater, Pennsylvania. The author or coauthor of over 110 journal articles, book chapters, and abstracts, and coauthor of one book, he is a member of the American Society for Microbiology, American Association of Immunologists, American Association of Virologists, and Infectious Diseases Society of America, among others. Dr. Six received the B.A. degree (1963) in chemistry from David Lipscomb College, Nashville, Tennessee, and the Ph.D. degree (1972) in microbiology from Vanderbilt University, Nashville, Tennessee.

Printed and bound by CPI Group (UK) Ltd, Croydon, CR0 4YY

17/10/2024

01775658-0002